DATE DUE

JE 02 '80	FE 28 '8		
AG 04 '8	AP 18 8		
OC 13 '	OC 24 '83		
NO 17 '8	O 21 '83		
DE 22 '8	MY 21 '8		
	DE 10 '8		
OC 26 '8	MR 04 '8		
NO 16 '8	FE 22 '88		
DE 14 '	MR 13 '9		
MR 08 '8	R 06		
MR 29 '8	MR 30 '00		
MY 10 '82			

The Overeaters

The Overeaters

Eating Styles and Personality

Jonathan Wise, M.D.

Susan Kierr Wise

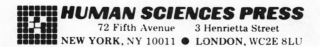

HUMAN SCIENCES PRESS
72 Fifth Avenue   3 Henrietta Street
NEW YORK, NY 10011 ● LONDON, WC2E 8LU

Copyright © 1979 by Human Sciences Press
72 Fifth Avenue, New York, New York 10011

Printed in the United States of America
9 987654321

Library of Congress Cataloging in Publication Date

Wise, Jonathan.
   The overeaters.

   Bibliography: p.
   Includes index.
   1. Obesity—Psychological aspects. I. Wise, Susan Kierr, joint author. II. Title.
RC552.025W57   616.3'98'019   79-719
ISBN 0-87705-405-3

To our children, Karren, Daniel, Seth, Alexander, and Sarah, without whom this book may have been written sooner.

Contents

1. AN INTRODUCTION   11

2. A MEDICAL VIEW OF THE OVEREATER

    Introduction   15
    Overeating and Obesity   16
    Diseases Leading to Overeating
      and/or Obesity   20
    "New" Disorders of Metabolism   27
    The Regulation of Appetite   34

3. THE FRIGHTENED OVEREATER:
    THE ORAL CLUSTER

    The Dynamics   44
    Harry: 800 Pounds and Deprived   47
    Dolly: The 25-year-old Baby   53

4. THE ANGRY OVEREATER:
    THE ANAL CLUSTER

    The Dynamics   58
    Ellen: The Cool, Calm, and
      Collected Binge Eater   69
    Martin: The Alienated Overeater   73
    A Letter from Marie   78
    Olga: The Depressed Pianist with
      an Alcoholic Mother   80
    Jack: The Angry Jogger with an
      Alcoholic Father   81

5. THE SEXUAL OVEREATER:
   THE GENITAL CLUSTER

   The Dynamics   86
   Rena: Being a Woman and Feeling
      Dirty   88
   Beth: The Infertile Overeater   92
   Lee: The Little Mom   94
   Dave: Being a Man   99
   Morris: The Little Phallus   101

6. THE ADOLESCENT-ONSET OVEREATER

   The Dynamics   106
   Bobbie: The 37-year-old Teenage
      Junk Food Addict   109
   Fusion and Rebellion   112

7. THE ADULT-ONSET OVEREATER

   The Dynamics   116
   Millie: Frustration in Marriage   117
   Kenneth: The Ex-Football Player   119
   Women in the Home   123
   Melissa: Failures and Regressions   125
   Julie: The Career Woman   128

8. SOCIETY AND THE OVEREATER

   Feast or Famine   134
   The Community   140
   Momism   142
   A Self-Fulfilling Prophecy: The
      Case of Michelle   146
   How We Feed Our Children   152
   How We View Obesity   154
   What We Can Do   155

9. MOVEMENT AS THERAPY

   The Instrument: The Body   157
   The Way It Worked for Olga and
      Martin   161

Action in the Treatment of Millie,
    Ellen, Rena, and Roger   163
Postures and Gestures: The Cases of
    Dolly and Nancy   170
Discovering What the Body Needs   174
Dealing with the Body-Image   176

10. TREATMENT

Oral Cluster   178
Anal Cluster   182
Genital Cluster   187
Adolescent-Onset Cluster   193
Adult-Onset Cluster   198
Social Factors   200

Notes   203

Index   211

1

An Introduction

*W*hen we commenced our private practices in endocrinology and dance therapy we were both struck by the inordinately high percentage of overweight individuals who came to us. Endocrinologists and dance therapists seem to attract people with weight problems. Many obese people feel that they have a glandular or hormonal problem and that if an endocrinologist can pinpoint the cause, their weight would go down once and for all. Furthermore, many overweight people have read that they do not move enough, that their lives are too sedentary. Consequently, they also tend to seek treatment from therapists trained in movement and dance.

Unfortunately, as we have found, the fields of endocrinology and dance therapy have not to date dealt with weight and eating problems adequately. As we explored the realm of psychology we found that this field too did not contribute satisfactorily to our understanding of the eating problems of individual patients. How then could we deal honestly and effectively with the increasing number of people who were seeking our help?

Traditionally, endocrinologists take a rather systematic approach to the obese patient. The physician first obtains a medical history, which evaluates the possibility of a known glandular disorder that might contribute to weight or eating problems. This history leads to a medical hypothesis, which is then tested in the laboratory whenever possible. For example, if the patient has symptoms which suggest a thyroid disorder, specific thyroid tests are ordered from the laboratory. If a woman is excessively hairy and has other symptoms suggesting an adrenal or ovarian problem, these glands are tested. Unfortunately, only a small percentage of patients has a known endocrinological disease. For most people, endocrinology can offer no explanation for their obesity.

Dance therapists have their own approach to problems involving weight and body image. Observing the movements, postures, and gestures of the patient, the therapist attempts to determine where in the body muscular tension is produced and repressed. The dance therapist, like the endocrinologist, attempts first to classify the individual's problem. Once that has been done, appropriate treatment can be suggested. The observations of the dance therapist frequently reveal needs and contradictions too complex to be cured by routine exercises.

It is our firm belief that people with weight problems cannot all be considered together. Overeaters must be classified systematically according to their unique problems. The development of such a system of classification requires knowledge in many fields. Information about both body and mind are needed, as well as about the interaction of the two, since for most overeating is the physical manifestation of an emotional problem.

In the study that follows, therefore, we have classified most overeaters according to their specific emotional problems. We have found that patients typically fall into certain categories according to these personality problems and have coined the term "clusters" to refer to a group of related problems. By classifying overeaters according to the oral, anal, or genital cluster, for example, we have established a diagnostic system that also implies a form of treatment tailored to the particular needs of such personality types.

Since eating is a central, early need, it is not surprising that it is closely tied to every person's emotional core. If a serious emotional problem arises at an early age, this may well be reflected in the person's later eating habits. Each cluster of overeaters is comprised of people whose conflicts arise at a particular critical stage of emotional development; such people would tend, therefore, to have certain personality traits and eating problems in common. By learning what these key traits are, we have been able to ask the right questions and to watch for revealing aspects of behavior and movement. Once we have some idea of the developmental stage in which a patient's problem is rooted, we can deal with the underlying issues instead of with superficial symptoms.

Erik Erikson, a leading figure in the field of psychoanalysis, has done important work in the classification and characterization of childhood development. We have found his approach very useful and have applied his descriptions of the critical stages of development to our own analysis of patients' eating patterns. When we applied Erikson's theories to our patients, we found that eating problems began to make sense as indicators of unresolved developmental conflicts. Our attempts at dealing with overeaters became less chaotic and rather more scientific. Consequently, we no longer floundered with our treatment.

The choice of a particular course of treatment, as the reader will see, followed the proper diagnosis of cluster. Instead of saying that all overweight people should go on the same diet, we now could say that each cluster of patients needed to be treated in a specific way and that certain underlying emotional problems had to be dealt with while treating the eating problem itself.

Unfortunately, the diagnosis of emotional problems is not as clear-cut as the diagnosis of physiological disease. No one of our patients belonged entirely to one developmental cluster. Unresolved problems arising during an early stage of development frequently carry over into later stages of life and cause further complications. Therefore, an adult may have an eating problem reflective of more than one cluster. Yet one cluster always seems to dominate the picture, and we have found it most useful in our treatment of patients to focus on the problems of the dominant cluster. Since the diagnosis of cluster clarifies the individual's particular emotional problems so well, it has become the cornerstone of our approach.

2

A Medical View of the Overeater

INTRODUCTION

In this chapter we will deal with the physiology of eating problems and with the medical causes of overeating. As will become evident, the majority of eating problems cannot now be expained by physiology alone. Current research and new findings all seem to indicate that emotional problems explain the eating habits of the majority of overeaters.

Many overeaters are unhappy. Their eating behavior is beyond their control. The physician or body therapist treating such people wants to know first whether or not the mechanisms controlling their appetite and weight are functioning normally. He or she must make the proper medical diagnosis. If the patient has a purely physiological disease or disorder, it must, of course, be assessed and treated.

Unfortunately, most professionals have trouble dealing with the overeater's cry for help. Information concerning normal eating patterns and appetite regulation is scattered and frequently too technical for those in clinical practice. In general, diseases which cause overeating have been poorly covered in the clinical literature. Diseases which affect the "burning" of food in the body itself are even more poorly understood.

People with weight problems sometimes suspect that they are not burning their food properly, that something is wrong with their "metabolism." They feel that they can gain weight even when they do not overeat.

Usually the professional shrugs off these remarks. He argues, perhaps out of ignorance: "You must eat a tremendous amount of food." The professional needs to know more about *normal* metabolism. He must know more about the disease of overeating. He must understand what can go wrong with metabolism and with the regulation of appetite.

The need to understand eating behavior is more imperative than ever before in our overweight society. More knowledge in this area would make the physician more effective and the public less apt to pursue faddish diets, outlandish theories, and magical cures.

Overeating and Obesity

When can a person conclude that his or her problem is overeating? After all, overeating frequently exists without ever becoming a serious problem—we all overeat at some time or other.

Stressful events may lead us to overeat. One young man overeats while studying for an exam, while another spends several days gorging due to an emotionally taxing family reunion or holiday season. For these brief periods of time such persons are overeaters.

Small children frequently go on food binges. Some seem to eat almost nothing for several days (or only small amounts of a favored food), then eat almost everything in sight for a day or two, trying new foods and consuming large quantities. Parents frequently become disturbed when their children go on these "diets," but it seems to be a quite natural pattern in the very young.

Early man's existence was also punctuated by periods of relative starvation and periods of binging. The hunter might go without food for an extended period of time and finally make a kill, resulting in binge eating. Thus, man's evolutionary past as well as childhood development bear witness to the wide daily fluctuations in food intake. These fluctuations have been dealt with beautifully by man's metabolic and hormonal processes, which govern mechanisms for feasting and fasting.

Some people get professional help because they are disturbed about the wide fluctuations in their food intake. We have seen many patients who are essentially nonobese but who are still concerned about their "eating problem." What bothers them is that at times they seem—for no apparent reason—to crave bread or ice cream or some other food and almost uncontrollably overeat. In order to prevent weight gain they go on a starvation diet for several days. Later they binge again.

Because such people are often disturbed by this cyclical pattern and would rather eat "like a normal person," they seek professional help. We believe these patients have an exaggerated notion of the normal process of intermittent overeating, since our own definition of a normal eater makes allowances for occasional binging.

If binging is not followed by periods of relatively low caloric intake, overeating will of course lead to weight gain. Persistent overeating without its opposite can be partially defined by a resultant obesity.

By contrast, we all probably know a few people who seem always to eat a tremendous amount of food but never become fat. We would say of such individuals that they are not binging or persistently overeating, since something tells them they need a great deal of food in order to maintain their weight. The disparity between their weight and their food intake can be explained by a very high caloric expenditure. It is quite obvious why such people expend so many calories. They are very active, and even when theoretically sitting still fidget, squirm, or otherwise make many small, restless movements. The combination of outright exercise and unconscious restless movement often explains why some people "burn" more calories than most.

Clearly, different activity patterns and habits result in varying weights for individuals whose food intake may be similar. An obese patient, when sitting across from a doctor's desk, tends to give his or her history with few body movements. The patient does little repositioning in the chair, and little else except the mouth seems to move. To some extent this depression of even basal activity is the result of an oral personality (discussed at length in the chapter on the oral cluster).

A fascinating study has been made by Rose and Williams which bears on our observations concerning the movements of obese patients.[1] They investigated twelve nonobese men who were roughly the same weight and age, but whose histories indicated greatly varied food intake. Some seemed to eat much more than others despite the fact that they weighed the same. Their basal metabolisms (which we will discuss in the next section of this chapter) were not significantly different. With forced exercise on a treadmill at a predetermined rate their energy expenditure seemed to be about the same. However, when they were allowed to do things at their own rate, major differences appeared. When told to walk, the men who ate a great deal walked at a faster rate and were more energetic, suggesting that they were habitually faster movers and burned more calories in general. The nonobese men who were less active ate less. Therefore, their weight remained within the normal range. If they had eaten as much as the big eaters, they would have been overeating relative to their energy output. Clearly, an innate mechanism was at work regulating their appetite.

In summary, the obese patient who denies the fact that he overeats is still an overeater because he eats too much relative to his caloric expenditure. The nonobese patient who burns fewer calories than normal appropriately adjusts his food intake by undereating. The mechanisms that regulate his appetite and therefore his food intake are normal. His eating habits are normal, and he does not overeat except on occasion. Hence, an overeater is one who is obese or one in whom the normal intermittent process of "feasting and fasting" is not operating correctly.

Much has been written in the medical literature in an attempt to define obesity. It is our belief that this is a rather futile effort, since normal weight depends largely upon the patient's health, pattern of activity, and general feeling of well-being. If a patient, for example, has diabetes mellitus and is also obese it is important that he lose weight. His weight problem may be quite mild, but because of his disease his obesity is of medical significance and must be treated. The trained football player, by contrast, may weigh twenty to thirty percent above his ideal weight, but it would be difficult to argue that he is truly obese since his muscle bulk is so tremendous. Therefore, such guidelines to weight as established in the Metropolitan Life Insurance tables are less than ideal in defining obesity.

Many patients complain of weight problems even though their weight is only five to ten percent above their so-called ideal weight. Indeed, they may have a real problem in that they have an excess amount of fat on one part of their body—thighs, hips, belly, etc. As far as they are concerned, they are "fat." This type of obesity could better be called localized obesity, but it is still a real problem and must be dealt with by the professional. Frequently, it has to be brought to the patient's attention that this type of fat distribution is common in his or her family. If a woman's face, arms, torso, and lower legs are quite thin, it seems to us best not to treat the localized fat deposit on her thighs. If she has a severe localized fat problem along with a mild generalized fat problem, then we consider the Metropolitan Life Insurance tables to have underestimated her true obesity. Simple localized obesity with no other evidence of a generalized fat problem should, we believe, not be deemed true obesity.

DISEASES LEADING TO OVEREATING AND/OR OBESITY

A reader might now say, "I know I am an unusual case. I do not sit still all day. I am energetic. I move my arms around when I talk. I am not a bump on a log. I do all of those things you accuse many of us of not doing. But I can't seem to lose weight when I diet. What's wrong with me?"

In our respective practices we have dealt with many obese patients who claim that they do not eat "that much." When they are put on a metabolic ward where their intake and output are strictly monitored, it is usually found that on the diet they claim they were adhering to, they lose weight. In fact, we have seen over and over again that on a 600-calorie diet obese individuals tend to lose weight faster than nonobese individuals. They have an especially rapid weight loss during the first week of dieting. This is due largely to fluid loss—obese persons tend to retain more fluid than the nonobese. On a low-calorie diet there tends to be a dramatic decrease in salt intake. Because of this decrease less fluid can be retained by the body and more is eliminated in the urine. Furthermore, there is strong evidence that a low-carbohydrate diet itself results in significant fluid loss. Since an obese person usually retains more fluid than a nonobese person, the amount of fluid he or she is able to lose while dieting is greater than for a nonobese individual.

Another reason why most obese patients lose weight more rapidly than nonobese patients on a metabolic ward is that they tend to have an accelerated basal metabolism. This fact contradicts the widely held myth that obese individuals have a sluggish metabolism. In order to correct and clarify this myth, let us first define and explain the term basal metabolism.

Even at rest the body is involved in innumerable activities simply to maintain body heat and to carry on basic involuntary processes. Basal metabolism provides the energy for this. What follows is a description of some of these processes at rest which require energy.

Energy derived from food or from the breakdown of the body's own tissues (called endogenous fuel) is stored in high-energy bonds, usually in a molecule of ATP. The energy from these bonds can be released under certain conditions and at times when the body requires it. When the body needs a great deal of energy, these ATP molecules are used at a faster rate. The body has various mechanisms which sense that this is happening and therefore signal the body to make more ATP. During such times more food or endogenous fuel is consumed (oxidized) to make ATP. At this point the so-called metabolism of the body is revved up. This kind of metabolism can be measured: we can estimate ATP production by measuring the amount of oxygen the patient consumes. By "burning" the fuel in oxygen, the oxygen is "used up" and becomes carbon dioxide and water. The higher the patient's metabolism, the less oxygen he will breathe out relative to the amount of oxygen he has just taken in. He is consuming more oxygen in his body.

If the patient eats a large meal, but does not require much energy at that particular time, he simply stores the food. Sugar, for example, can be stored as glycogen. However, when he is using up his ATP or high-energy bonds, this glycogen will be broken down in order to supply the body with more ATP. Oxygen consumption increases, the endogenous fuels are broken down, and energy is supplied at the right time and place within the body.

As we have stated, the body is in a state of dynamic flux even when it is at rest. Energy is needed to maintain the steady state. Much of this activity takes place in the cells of the body.

The cell membrane separates the internal environment of the cell from the fluid that bathes the cell. The internal contents of the cell differ from this external or extracellular fluid. The cell's ability to perform various functions and activities depends upon this biochemical environment; the amount of sodium, potassium, and other ions within the cell are particularly critical. A very active energy-requiring metabolic process occurs at the cell membrane which controls this ionic equilibrium between intracellular and extracellular fluid. The process is especially active in the kidney, where ions are actively transported to and from the urine-to-be into and out of the cells of the kidney. This active transport requires energy. In fact, it has been estimated that over one-half of the basal metabolism is involved in this membrane transport of ions throughout the body.

Basal metabolism supplies the brain with energy or ATP. Involuntary movements of muscle such as those of the gut, the diaphragm, and the heart require continual energy production. New cells are constantly being made and energy is needed for this process. The body is teeming with activity even at rest.

Since obese individuals have a larger body surface than lean people, there is more area for this activity to go on. More ions must be transported. Since more tissue is present, more tissue and fluid must be maintained in a steady state. If other conditions are held constant, obese individuals have a higher basal energy expenditure than nonobese individuals. This fact is confirmed by the finding that the oxygen consumption of an obese patient at rest is greater than that of a lean patient. As we have already explained, this oxygen consumption reflects the energy expenditure or the amount of ATP being produced within the body.

Why, the reader may wonder, if the "metabolism" of obese patients who are otherwise healthy and normal is greater than the metabolism of nonobese patients, is it not considered overactive? The answer is simple: the BMR or basal metabolic rate is derived from the patient's oxygen consumption and is calculated by dividing the oxygen consumed by the patient's weight. The more the patient weighs, the more is divided into the oxygen consumption. An extreme example of this occurs when one compares the measurement of metabolism in mice and elephants—even though, of course, the absolute metabolism of an elephant is much greater than that of a mouse. Similarly, the BMR of obese and lean persons can be compared: the absolute metabolism of an otherwise healthy obese person will always be greater than that of the lean person.

Of course, if an obese person has a physiologically induced metabolic problem, his or her metabolism can be termed relatively "sluggish." He or she may require less ATP to keep the body functioning and, hence, may burn less food to produce the ATP. More of the food is then stored as fat or glycogen, waiting to be called upon as an energy source in the future. The person gains weight as a consequence.

Specifically, hypothyroidism (underactive thyroid) is one condition that can produce a sluggish metabolism. When a patient with this condition takes thyroid hormone in pill form, his or her oxygen consumption or "metabolism" is increased. There are several reasons for this increase.

The administration of thyroid hormone to the hypothyroid child results in a growth spurt. Until the thyroid pill is given to the child, his or her growth is usually quite retarded. Growth requires ATP since bone, muscle, protein, fat, and cell production in general require energy. For the hypothyroid adult who has stopped growing, the administration of thyroid hormone also stimulates the production of protein. Energy or ATP is required, and until the patient receives the thyroid pill, he or she produces and breaks down less protein than normal. Similarly, administration of thyroid hormone stimulates the production and breakdown of fat. In effect, it accelerates the normal need of the body to revitalize itself by breaking down "old" fat and protein and making "new" fat and protein.

Thyroid hormone increases oxygen consumption or metabolism in other ways. However, most of these mechanisms are still poorly understood. The interested reader is referred to the notes at the end of this chapter for sources providing a more extensive discussion of such mechanisms.[2,3]

A physician will routinely look for a thyroid "condition" when he or she is evaluating the causes of obesity in a patient. Unfortunately, this search almost always proves fruitless. When people develop an underactive thyroid, there is usually a decrease in their appetite and, consequently, in their food intake. Therefore, they tend to have only a very mild increase in fat. Much of their weight gain is due to fluid retention. When they are treated with thyroid pills, they do lose weight quickly at first, but this weight loss is largely fluid loss.

The physician will also look for an overactive adrenal gland in an obese person. Patients with this problem produce too many steroids. Their bodies are exposed to high levels of steroid and this exposure causes the weight gain. Also some patients are being given steroid pills to treat other problems such as arthritis or asthma. These patients, receiving a steroid, tend to get fat. Cortisone, a well-known steroid, can produce weight gain.

An excess of steroids can be detected by the peculiar distribution of fat on the patient's body. The torso, for example, gets fat and bears reddish stretch marks, while the arms and legs stay relatively thin. Muscles waste away to some degree because the glucocorticoids speed up the breakdown of body protein.

Even though steroids decrease muscle bulk relative to fat bulk, the primary problem as far as weight gain is concerned is due to overeating. Steroids seem to stimulate the appetite, at times making it quite ravenous. The buildup of fat is, therefore, largely the result of overeating.

True diseases of the adrenal gland are very rare, but the use of steroid medications is now common. These patients receiving steroids must be understood by the professional and not simply scolded for overeating.

In the disease called Stein-Leventhal Syndrome the ovaries secrete too many steroids. These steroids are similar in structure to those produced by the adrenal gland. It is probable that they also stimulate the appetite and, hence, cause obesity. These ovarian hormones also produce too much hair. Obese women who have very irregular periods and considerable body hair may be suffering from Stein-Leventhal Syndrome. This condition is relatively common, and can now be diagnosed and treated successfully.

Another glandular disorder that may result in overeating is due to an insulin-secreting tumor involving the pancreas. This tumor is called an insulinoma. People with such tumors sometimes—though rarely—get obese. Because these tumors secrete an excessive amount of insulin, the insulin drives the sugar from the blood into the cells. The result frequently is low blood sugar, which in turn causes overeating.

Insulin-secreting tumors put insulin into the blood stream no matter if there is a need for it or not. Hence, when the blood sugar starts to drop during fasting, insulin still goes into the blood stream and lowers the blood sugar to very low levels. By contrast, when a normal person fasts, insulin levels in the blood drop to very low levels so that the blood sugar itself is never dangerously low. (As we shall see later in this chapter, the blood sugar seems to be an important factor in the regulation of the brain's appetite center.) With their very low blood sugars, patients with this very rare disease do find that they eat excessively. In this way they are able to avoid the dangerous condition fasting might produce in their bodies or at least to minimize episodes of low blood sugar. Unfortunately, the price they pay is weight gain.

Some diabetics on insulin have repeated insulin "reactions." During a reaction the blood sugar level is too low. It is unusual for a patient to have repeated insulin reactions day after day without consulting a physician or lowering his insulin dose himself. But if he continued to take too much insulin, his situation would be similar to the patient with an insulin-secreting tumor: he would overeat and gain weight.

It is often said that many people overeat because they have repeated attacks of low blood sugar. This notion is attractive to some obese patients since they can attribute their eating behavior to a known medical problem and can, therefore, expect a readily available, rather effortless, and rapid cure. In reality, however, there is no evidence that obese individuals while fasting tend to develop low blood sugars more often than lean people. That is to say, when an overweight person diets his blood sugar does not fall too low, thus causing him to break his diet. In fact, studies have shown that obese patients maintain higher blood sugar levels after a fast than nonobese patients. (A condition does exist in which low blood sugar develops three to five hours after eating, not during a fast. However, there is no scientific evidence to support the theory that this condition plays a genuine role in the development of obesity.)

In summary, we have discussed in this section diseases

that can result in overeating and obesity. In the next section we will speculate on "diseases" which are less clearcut but which may affect metabolism and/or eating behavior.

"New" Disorders of Metabolism

New and still evolving material related to metabolism and obesity is continually being presented in the medical literature. Since this information is by its very nature speculative and allows no final conclusions from researchers, we wish to stress—for professional and layman alike—the necessity for accepting scientific ambiguities. Simple-minded dogmas are neither tenable nor useful.

We know, first of all, that hormones other than thyroid can have an effect on metabolism. However, whether or not these other hormones play a role in the development of obesity is not known. The two groups of hormones that have been implicated are the catecholamines and growth hormones.

The catecholamines are epinephrine (adrenalin) and norepinephrine. In response to stress, these hormones are released into the blood stream from the adrenal gland and sympathetic nerve endings. Sweating occurs; the pupils dilate; the heart beats faster; sugar is released from the liver into the blood stream; more blood flows into the muscles as metabolism accelerates. All of these effects, and many more, provide the body with an overall response which helps it to survive stress.

The catecholamines, then, accelerate metabolism in order to provide the ATP which is acutely needed to combat stress. This is a healthy human response. There exists, however, a well-studied disease in which an excessive amount of these hormones is produced and secreted into the blood stream. This is caused by a tumor called a pheochromocytoma. Persons with such tumors have uncontrollable episodes which mimic all of the changes that occur during severe stress, including, of course, an accelerated metabolism. Some of these episodes may be protracted, causing the metabolism to be accelerated for relatively long periods of time. Appetite decreases, further contributing to weight loss. Since the metabolism may also be accelerated when the thyroid gland is overactive, a pheochromocytoma can be confused with a thyroid condition.

The ingestion of amphetamines can also result in a stressful state similar to that induced by a pheochromocytoma. Amphetamines cause a release of catecholamines from their storage sites in nerve endings. The nerve endings, which activate the release of these hormones, are part of the sympathetic nervous system. When the hormones are released from their storage sites, they can act on their target sites, such as the heart, causing a rapid heartbeat, perspiration, and accelerated metabolism. Amphetamines, like an overactive thyroid gland and a pheochromocytoma, can make one irritable and shaky. More calories are burned up when movements quicken, and appetite decreases.

In summary, excessive stimulation of the sympathetic nervous system, either from a pheochromocytoma or from amphetamines, results in an accelerated metabolism, an increase of movements at so-called rest, and a depressed appetite. These three factors in turn result in weight loss. The sympathetic nervous system, therefore, may well be central in weight control. (The importance of this fact will be discussed later when we deal with appetite regulation.)

We turn now to the question of whether a disease exists in cases where these catecholamines are decreased and the patient gains weight. Though our position may change with further research in the field, we believe now that some people who weigh more than their eating habits would attest to show such evidence of a depressed sympathetic nervous system.

The ideal way to investigate the sympathetic nervous

system in an obese patient is to evaluate his or her sympathetic response under stress. For example, if one were only to estimate his or her catecholamine production while at rest, one would know nothing about the patient's ability to have a vigorous sympathetic response. Stress is necessary in order to test the reserve capacity of the sympathetic nervous system. Unfortunately, few experiments are conducted under stress. Secondly, it is difficult to even estimate the activity of the sympathetic nervous system. Nerves that release catecholamines are in close contact with target organs, such as the heart. The hormone, therefore, is released locally, and most of it is broken down by enzymes at these local sites. Because of this, relatively little norepinephrine can be measured in the blood and urine and one wonders how closely this measurement reflects the actual amount of hormone that was present at the local site of action. Despite these reservations, we will cite the data currently available in evaluating the sympathetic nervous system under stress.

Exposure to cold is stressful to the body, which reacts by an increase in metabolism. This rise in metabolism would appear to be appropriate, since in a cold environment more heat is needed to maintain the body temperature at the normal 98.6. In order to supply heat more fuel must be burned up or metabolized by the body. Yet what tells the body to accelerate metabolism under this stressful condition? It has been shown that the sympathetic nervous system is shifted into a higher gear under conditions of cooling. It seems likely, then, that the sympathetic nervous system plays a central role in signaling the body to accelerate its metabolism.

Quaade has studied increases in metabolism in response to cooling in both obese and lean subjects by measuring oxygen consumption as a reflection of metabolism.[4] During his experiments, conducted under cold conditions, lean subjects showed a 33 percent rise in oxygen consumption while obese subjects experienced only an 11 percent rise. Obviously, the obese patients had much better insulation in the form of fat and, as a result, required less of a rise in metabolism to maintain normal body temperature. Cold exposure for them was less stressful and, therefore, they did not need to turn their sympathetic nervous system into such high gear.

However—a much more surprising statistic—patients who denied overeating had even lower rises in their oxygen consumption on exposure to cold. These subjects included both lean and obese patients. The lean subjects who ate relatively small amounts of food showed only a 10 percent rise in their oxygen consumption. By comparison, the lean overeaters showed a 41 percent rise in their oxygen consumption. The obese subjects who claimed that they ate relatively small amounts of food experienced only a 2.5 percent rise in their oxygen consumption, while the obese overeaters had a 37 percent rise in their oxygen consumption. Quaade's study suggests, therefore, that some people cannot shift their sympathetic nervous system into high gear in response to the stress of cooling. As we shall see, these same people may have a generalized depression of their sympathetic nervous system, their metabolism being not very responsive to stress.

Obviously, every individual has a certain ability to accelerate his or her metabolism under stressful conditions. Some people have an average ability. More than likely most people are clustered near this average, and only a relatively few people are on the extreme ends of the continuum. Those few have a very unresponsive sympathetic nervous system and tend to become obese. They often seek help, and it is most unfortunate that many professionals cannot really differentiate them from the obese people who simply overeat.

By examining the sympathetic nervous system during the stress caused by overeating, Young and Landsberg have very recently explained (to our satisfaction) the phenomenon of diet-induced thermogenesis.[5] In this condition the body increases its heat production after overeating. Their experiments with animals have shown that a catecholamine in the heart increases with overeating. Interestingly enough, a few studies have shown that some obese people do not increase their heat production after overeating. Apparently these patients do not burn up as well as they should some of the excess calories consumed by overeating. Given Young and Landsburg's research, we would postulate that such persons have a sympathetic nervous system which is relatively insensitive to the stimulus of overeating. We would also postulate that these same people have a sympathetic nervous system which is relatively unresponsive to the stress stimulus of cooling.

The concept of diet-induced thermogenesis requires further explanation. Miller and Mumford found that heat production after overeating increased in proportion to the size of the meal.[6] When subjects were exercised after a heavy meal, their heat production increased even more. In other words, with exercise there was an even greater dissipation of excess calories. This data lends credence to the old wives' tale that one should not go to sleep shortly after a big meal because much of the meal will be converted into fat.

Diet-induced thermogenesis may explain, at least in part, why nonobese subjects when force-fed do not gain the expected amount of weight. Specifically, if a normal person is given an extra 4,000 calories per day he or she gains less than 75 percent of what one would predict from the fact that about 3,500 calories equal approximately one pound of weight gain. Although studies have not been done as yet, it is possible that some obese subjects when given these extra calories gain closer to 100 percent of what one would predict from their calorie excess. If our theory is correct, one might also anticipate that these subjects would have a relatively unresponsive sympathetic nervous system.

However, the ultimate significance of diet-induced thermogenesis and its effect on weight gain with overfeeding is still far from clear. Studies have not yet been done with subjects who are exercised after overfeeding. Under these conditions, one might predict, from what we discussed above, a far greater dissipation of calories. Variations in exercise after overfeeding may explain the results obtained in some experiments where diet-induced thermogenesis seemed to be of little significance.

Teleologically, diet-induced thermogenesis due to the activation of the sympathetic nervous system is an intriguing concept. When early man killed an animal, he would overeat, increase his catecholamines, or sympathetic nervous system, and, as a result, increase his heat production. He could then fall asleep soundly and stay relatively warm without as much protection from the elements, i.e., cold. Some of his excess calories would be dissipated, and he would not be prone to gaining much weight. His great physical activity insured that even more calories would be dissipated, thus preventing him from becoming obese and sluggish—dangerous conditions for the primitive hunter. Between kills he would enter a state of relative starvation in which diet-induced thermogenesis would not be operative, and he would lose weight more slowly.

In summary, the sympathetic nervous system seems to be an important factor in the regulation of man's metabolism and in the regulation of overeating. As we shall see, these same catecholamines released by the sympathetic nervous system are also crucial in the regulation of appetite at the level of the brain. In extreme and probably rare cases, individuals might have sympathetic nervous systems which are so unresponsive to stress that they might have difficulty losing weight even on a relatively strict diet. Convenient tests should therefore be devised to evaluate an individual's response to stress.

As mentioned, growth hormone can also affect the ability to burn calories. Growth hormone is released from the pituitary gland in response to many stimuli. Low blood sugar, sleep, and certain amino acids are a few of the known stimuli which cause an elevation of growth hormone in the blood. It has been clearly shown that obesity itself inhibits the rise in growth hormone in response to these stimuli. If one were to force-feed a thin individual to the point of obesity, that individual would develop a reduced growth hormone response to such stimuli.[7]

Patients given an injection of growth hormone increase their oxygen consumption, since their metabolism has been accelerated. Growth hormone also has an effect on fat tissue: it causes more body fat to be broken down, which can then be utilized as fuel by the body. However, this effect on fat would not alone result in weight loss, since it simply diverts the metabolism more to fat and less to other fuels, such as protein. Nevertheless, growth hormone's effect on oxygen consumption may in turn produce some effect on weight loss.[8]

Certain obese patients have a blunted growth hormone response. Since this hormone accelerates metabolism, it is conceivable that a relative lack of it plays some role in maintaining obesity when it develops. However, we must emphasize that under normal conditions growth hormone levels in the blood are quite low. These levels are in sharp contrast to the high blood levels that result from the injection of growth hormone into the body or under such severe conditions as low blood sugar. Normally, when growth hormone levels are low, the hormone has only a very slight effect on oxygen consumption. At these relatively low levels, growth hormone variations between people would appear to be of little importance in maintaining obesity.

Like certain obese patients, lean subjects who become obese after being force-fed have the same blunted growth hormone responses. But once the forced feeding is stopped, they lose weight rapidly. In addition, when a normally obese patient loses weight his growth hormone responses return to normal.[9] Therefore, if he or she regains weight, that gain cannot be blamed on a "sluggish" metabolism due to decrease of growth hormone.

In conclusion, the growth hormone "problem" in obesity is nothing like the sympathetic nervous system "problem." The former is secondary to obesity, the reduced response of growth hormone being instead a consequence of obesity. The sympathetic nervous system "problem" seems to affect only a certain number of obese and nonobese patients. We postulate that these patients, whether obese or lean, have to watch their weight and food intake more closely than the average person. Their condition is not a consequence of obesity, but rather a primary problem. We further postulate that such patients may well have a normal basal or "resting" metabolism and that only under conditions of stress is it found to be "sluggish." The idea of an underactive sympathetic nervous system in relation to the problem of overweight is very intriguing, but it must be remembered that theories involving it are still quite speculative.

THE REGULATION OF APPETITE

The control of appetite is a very complex subject, as recent information attests. We hope here to extract and clarify the aspects of this topic which have the greatest relevance to our understanding of overeating.

The primary seat of appetite regulation is in the ancient or lower brain of man, called the hypothalamus. There are two centers of appetite control in this part of the brain: destruction of one center results in obesity, while destruction of the other results in loss of appetite and severe emaciation. One center governs the sense of fullness or satiation and the other transmits feelings of hunger.

Many nerve endings feed into the satiety and hunger centers of the hypothalamus. These endings release chemicals called neurotransmitters which tell the centers what is going on elsewhere in the body. For example, if the upper brain is stimulated by a large variety of tasty food in a supermarket, messages are transmitted from the upper brain down to the nerve endings in the hypothalamus. Neurotransmitters are released from the nerve endings in the hypothalamus in response to the electrical impulse or message from the upper to lower brain. These neurotransmitters then stimulate the hunger center. The hunger center in turn stimulates the mouth to salivate and, in other ways, creates the "feeling" of hunger. The individual may then buy some of the stimulating food.

What seems particularly essential to us is the fact that neurotransmitters are the mediators of hunger or satiation. In other words, they mediate between the "electrical" input into the hypothalamus and its response. Drugs or experimental conditions which have the capacity to directly release these mediators can also directly stimulate or depress the appetite. Once depleted, the hypothalamus cannot receive a proper message to eat or not to eat. The stomach full of food might still send a message to the center of satiation in the hypothalamus, but the concentration of the chemical or neurotransmitter that mediates the message would be low. Thus the satiation center would not receive a "correct" message, since the feeling of a full stomach would never be perceived normally and eating would continue beyond normal limits.

Certain conditions and diseases are known to effect derangements in the release and/or concentration of neurotransmitters. There are probably other disease states as yet unknown to medical science which can also interfere with these neurotransmitters, resulting in excessive hunger or in an inability to perceive satiety and, hence, causing overeating and subsequent obesity.

One such speculative disease which could result in overeating may be the condition in which the release of one very important group of neurotransmitters, the catecholamines, is depressed. Catecholamines are normally released from nerve endings in the hypothalamus in response to certain messages. If the "electrical" message were to get to the hypothalamus but the catecholamines were not released properly, the final message might then be distorted and interpreted incorrectly. Some people, as we mentioned earlier, appear to have a depression of catecholamine release elsewhere, namely in the sympathetic nervous system. We postulated that those people would have a blunted metabolism under stress. Could these same individuals have the same sort of problem with catecholamine release in another part of their bodies, i.e., the hypothalamus? This possibility definitely exists, and it is intriguing to speculate on it. Further research in this area is necessary, but already known facts lend credence to this theory.

Experiments have shown that the center of satiation can be stimulated by implanting electrodes in a specific area of the hypothalamus called the ventromedial nucleus. When these electrodes give off a small current of electricity in the area, there is an increase in the activity of the sympathetic nervous system in the body.[10] These experiments have been done only in lower animals thus far, but the implication is clear: an appetite-regulating area in the brain seems to be closely linked to the regulation of the body's metabolism via the sympathetic nervous system. If something goes awry with the appetite center, the sympathetic nervous system may have a blunted response to overeating or to stress in general. These findings suggest that catecholamines released in the hypothalamus by electrical stimulation are somehow connected to catecholamines released elsewhere in the body via the sympathetic nervous system. Studies have in fact been done in animals wherein catecholamines were injected directly into the appetite centers of the brain. These injected catecholamines, when they came into direct contact with the centers of hunger or satiation, caused changes in food intake.[11]

Amphetamines are known to stimulate the release of norepinephrine, an important catecholamine, from the endings of sympathetic nerve fibers in the brain. Since we know that amphetamines decrease appetite, it becomes obvious that such drugs work by increasing the neurotransmitter norepinephrine in the area of appetite regulation. Therefore, by increasing catecholamines in certain ways, one can depress appetite. This fact lends further credence to the theory that overeating can result from a defect in the release of one important group of neurotransmitters, the catecholamines.

At this point the overeater may conclude: "Here is my trouble! My sympathetic nerve endings do not release catecholamines as well as they should. So my metabolism does not increase under stress and my appetite center is thrown out of kilter. I'll just take an amphetamine, which will increase my catecholamines. My metabolism and my appetite regulation may then be better."

Such a conclusion, while tempting, is not only simplistic but also dangerous and the result would be disappointing. If a problem with sympathetic responsiveness does exist, it is a problem of degree and not absolute. The whole population could be plotted on a graph according to their degree of sympathetic responsiveness. Most persons would be near the middle of the graph and only a few would be at the extremes. In other words, only a very few would have an overly responsive or unresponsive sympathetic nervous system.

Since everyone is at a different point on the graph, it would be impossible to even attempt to rectify a faulty degree of responsiveness with pills. And if an ideal drug existed, what would the correct dosage be for a specific individual? We cannot expect miraculous cures even if we were to fully understand this part of our biology. As we stated earlier, medicine will never be able to cure overeating and obesity by understanding one biological problem alone.

Just as it is tempting to hope that a simple cause and effect will eventually be found for overeating, so too it is easy to give into despair when this fails to appear. But as we go on to describe the complexities of appetite control, it will be seen that an intricate system of control has indeed developed throughout mankind's evolution. Rather than despairing about dysfunctions in the system, we might marvel at the machinery of our body chemistry even with its imperfections.

A very finely tuned and sensitive piece of machinery regulates appetite. Information concerning changes in the condition of the body is fed into this machinery. For example, when a diabetic injects too much insulin into his or her body, there is a drop in blood sugar. In order to maintain the condition of stability (homeostasis) in the body's many systems, this drop in blood sugar must be countered by a response. Since the body must maintain a steady internal environment for good health, it must return the blood sugar to normal. Several events occur which allow this to happen. For example, a hormone called glucagon is released into the blood stream when there is such a drop in blood sugar. This event encourages the release of sugar from the liver into the blood stream where it is needed. More pertinent to our discussion, the machinery dealing with hunger is activated. The diabetic craves sugar, eats it, and brings his body back to the steady state.

Appetite regulation is crucial in maintaining homeostasis in other ways. If an animal gains a certain amount of unnecessary weight, its appetite center, by some unknown mechanism, senses this and consequently depresses its appetite. If rats were force-fed to the point of obesity and later were left alone to eat whatever they wanted, they would eat very little until they returned to their original weight. Homeostasis would thereby be regained. Clearly, their original weight has survival value. Simply stated, an overweight rat runs more slowly and is more easily caught by a lean, hungry cat.

Scientists studying obesity have been impressed with the degree to which appetite regulation is sensitive to changes in blood sugar and body weight or fat. They have termed glucostat that part of the appetite regulation center which is sensitive to changes in blood sugar and lipostat that part sensitive to changes in the size of fat cells (the latter closely reflects weight gain or total body fat).[12,13]

In order to understand the idea of a lipostat and what it may mean to the overeater, we must refer to the work of Hirsch and his colleagues. They and others found that after a certain age an individual who gains weight simply increases the size of his fat cells.[14,15] The actual number of fat cells stays fixed despite further weight gain. There are, however, a few critical periods in earlier life when an individual's weight gain is accompanied by an increase in the number as well as the size of fat cells. Specifically, persons who gain a great deal of weight and become obese in early childhood or early adolescence have more fat cells than individuals who become obese in adult life. Those with adult-onset obesity simply develop larger fat cells; the number of such cells stays the same. The number of fat cells is determined at crucial points in early life and does not waver thereafter. Once a child develops more fat cells than normal, he or she cannot really decrease that number even by losing weight later on in life.

Recently Hirsch and his colleagues reported on a series of experiments with rats.[16] In one study fat tissue—and therefore fat cells—were surgically removed from one group of rats. This group and another group which did not have the surgery were then fed a fattening diet. Both the surgical and nonsurgical group gained weight, but the surgical group gained less weight. When the size of fat cells was measured after the weight gain, the two groups were seen to have the same cell size. The surgical group gained less weight because they ate less. In a sense they had fewer fat cells to "feed"; therefore, their fat cells became fatter at the same rate as the nonsurgical group despite the fact that they ate less. The rate of increase in the size of fat cells seemed to control the intake of food. Ultimately, however, the number of fat cells that had to be "fed" determined how large those cells would become if given a certain amount of food. Regulation of weight in these rats was therefore dictated by the number of fat cells in the body. Simply stated, rats with fewer initial fat cells have fewer cells to "feed," which in turn causes them to eat less and to remain thinner.

Similarly, individuals with more fat cells to begin with have more cells to feed, therefore eat more and gain more weight. How is the message sent from the fat cell to the lipostat in the hypothalamus? We do not know. It would be a real breakthrough if, for example, a chemical substance were to be found which could act as this mediator. Not only would the lipostat theory gain further credence, but something could possibly be done about lowering this mediator through chemical means. Then the obese person who has too many fat cells would not have an appetite driven by his "hungry" fat cells.

Many people gain weight and become truly obese at times other than those critical periods when the number of fat cells is determined. Therefore, there is no possibility that their appetite is driven by hungry fat cells. The lipostat mechanism does not explain their excessive appetites. Nor, except in rare instances, does the glucostat mechanism explain the excessive appetite of most overweight people. As we have already stated, one rarely finds recurrent low blood sugar with resultant obesity. Mechanisms other than the lipostat and glucostat have been postulated, but none of them adequately explain why most obese people overeat. The reader who wishes to know more about these mechanisms can read the information contained in references cited at the end of this chapter.[17,18]

Why are the mechanisms controlling appetite regulation not working normally in these overeaters? Why do they not seem to listen to these appetite regulators? When the fat cell starts to grow in size, the lipostat mechanism should put a brake on food intake. But the overeater continues to overeat, apparently not responding to his lipostat.

Studies by Campbell and others have shown that obese subjects, unlike lean subjects, have trouble adjusting their food intake according to changes in the caloric content of their food.[19] Obese and lean subjects were both fed a liquid formula. After a certain period of time, the caloric content of the formula was reduced without changing its consistency or taste. The appetite centers of the lean subjects "sensed" this change much better than those of the obese subjects. They began to drink more of the liquid so that they tended to consume the same number of calories as before. By contrast, the obese subjects did not increase their intake so consistently. They lost weight. Again we see that the overeater has a defect in his or her appetite regulation mechanism.

Because overeaters do not "listen" to these internal mechanisms governing appetite control, they become more vulnerable to external mechanisms of appetite regulation. Even if their bodies are picking up internal cues, they do not respond to the messages properly. The external cues alone tend to tell them when and how much to eat.

We are all bombarded with external stimuli which tell us that we would love to savor this creamy treat or that tasty morsel. The obese person, who is already highly vulnerable to external cues in the regulation of his or her appetite, is especially apt to succumb to the barrage of food advertisements in stores and media alike. The commercialism of our society has magnified this person's problem. The lean individual, who regulates his appetite more according to the internal mechanisms we have just discussed, is partly protected from this onslaught of commercialism. Unfortunately, the individual who can be harmed the most by these eating suggestions is also the most sensitive to external cues.

Schacter's experiments substantiate the theory that obese people are more vulnerable to external cues.[20,21] In one experiment, for example, he changed the time on the clock in the room where obese and nonobese individuals had a ready supply of food. If he moved the clock ahead by two hours, the obese people tended to eat when the clock read six o'clock even though it was only four o'clock. The nonobese people tended to wait, so to speak, until their appetite centers told them that they were hungry. They were less vulnerable to the external stimulus of a clock.

Because obese patients are so vulnerable to external stimuli, they are also quite amenable to a form of therapy called behavior modification. By changing the stimuli in their environment, they can often change their eating behavior. By removing a wide variety of goods from their environment, for instance, they can adhere to a diet more easily. By staying away from supermarkets, they cannot see and cannot therefore be stimulated by the attractive packaging on high-calorie products. By using only one dish or bowl to eat from, they will not be confronted by a dessert dish which stimulates their appetite for something sweet.

Notwithstanding the frequently successful application of behavioral therapy in the short-term treatment of obesity, superficial modifications in eating habits and environmental manipulation are, in our opinion, never long-range solutions to the problems faced by overweight individuals. If there is one main thesis in this book, it is the following: most overeaters overeat for emotional reasons. Whenever overeating is used to suppress feelings and to deal with inner conflicts, the individual is not listening to his glucostat, lipostat, or any other part of his appetite regulation center. It seems reasonable to suppose that eventually such a person becomes quite insensitive to his appetite center, which in time is likely to atrophy from disuse. Thus internal stimuli or cues come to play an increasingly minor role in his appetite regulation, leaving the person vulnerable to external cues. Initially, however, the problem developed from within. Therefore, to truly treat the problem, one must deal with the inner conflict, whether it be primarily oral, anal, genital, etc. The ensuing chapters will discuss each of these conflicts in turn.

Behavior modification for the treatment of obesity is largely a regulation of external cues in an attempt to replace the individual's lost internal cues which would normally guide him to eat less. However, when an emotional situation arises which aggravates the basic eating conflict, this type of treatment readily falls apart as the overeater resumes his old behavior. If the overeater's emotional conflict can be healed, he may with time regain his internal mechanisms of appetite regulation. This healing may take years of psychotherapy. Until then the overeater must also rely on external forms of control, i.e., a diet, as well as suitable techniques of behavior modification.

3

The Frightened
Overeater
The Oral Cluster

THE DYNAMICS

*I*n our efforts to understand people who suffer from obesity, we have identified one group of overeaters who were caught in a frightening trap that began for them in early infancy, when they were in the oral stage of development. These people appear to have certain personality and eating characteristics in common. Patients belonging to the oral cluster require a form of treatment which is different from that for patients belonging to other clusters. Their prognosis is also different and somewhat less secure, since they have carried the very earliest—the oral— problems with them through all subsequent periods of growth. They are usually the most difficult patients to treat.

We have concentrated our own analysis of this stage on those patients who have presented themselves to us with both oral personality traits and persistent eating problems. By exploring their case histories, we have gained useful insights into the oral stage of development. It is through them that we have evolved the concept of an oral cluster of overeaters, and this has meant that we have been able to treat such people with clearer understanding and greater success than might otherwise have been possible.

It is essential that we know some of the previous work done in the field of psychology as it relates to the oral personality. Freud and Erikson, among others, have shown that either excessive satisfaction or excessive frustration at this earliest stage of childhood frequently results in particular problems and personality traits in adulthood.[1,2,3,4] The oral personality has experienced both extremes in early childhood. When dealing with this type of overeater, therefore, we must investigate early childhood conditions. His or her early relationship with the mother, or mother figure, is crucial, since the mother is central to the newborn. Above all, the mother is the key to understanding the patient belonging to the oral cluster.

Before birth, the child is one with the mother. This fusion, or symbiosis, can never be repeated outside the womb. After birth, it is totally dependent on the supplies it receives from the mother and does not at first even have an awareness of physical separation from her. The infant does not know where its body begins and ends, does not differentiate between what it feels and what the world feels. That is, when a newborn is hungry, it experiences the whole world as being hungry. If it is cold or wet or uncomfortable, the world is so experienced.

Ideally, early maternal care provides the infant with a world that is basically full, warm, and comfortable. If the mother is not able to provide this environment with some consistency, the child's separation from her is experienced as quite fearful. If the infant senses a trustworthy responsiveness in maternal care, then gradual separation does not seem as frightening. If no early feeling of safety has been established, then the issues of separation and safety haunt the child and later the adult.

Much of the affect and trust between mother and child during the earliest period of development revolves around food. The mother's warmth is initially related to the breast and/or bottle. The child feels her closeness, cradled and rocked in her arms, and so develops a basic trust in the mother's supplies. Feeding is one of the most central factors in the development of this positive intimacy.

It comes as no surprise, therefore, that if the foundation of this relationship is faulty, the child will be subjected to inadequate or disruptive, inconsistent supplies. Later in life, repeated attempts are made to relive some aspects of early maternal care in an effort to make it more adequate. One way of doing this is by overeating to the point of obesity. The overeating pattern becomes compulsive, a vain attempt to find adequate nurturance from a source that can be trusted.

Because all desires center around the mouth and both tensions and satisfactions are experienced through the mouth, the early months of life are referred to as the oral stage. If during this stage the child receives food when it experiences hunger, it learns that there is no devastating urgency to being hungry. If the tension produced by hunger is consistently relieved by the satisfaction of fullness, the child can trust its world. But if it is continually frustrated, it never really loses this frightened sense of urgency—the urgency of hunger or tension. As adults, they may find themselves still unable to tolerate even moderate tension, since it has become confused with a feeling of hunger. They could never trust that their infant needs would be met, and as adults have still not developed a real trust in their environment. Since their mothers could never really be trusted, they never really came to trust their own ability to get what they wanted. Food and supplies in general seem tenuous, as if they may disappear at any time. The need for supplies seems desperate and immediate, and postponement of gratification virtually intolerable.

The oral person's self-esteem, then, is dependent on getting food and supplies for warmth, comfort, and safety. This person has trouble trusting either his environment or his own resources. Such a person tends always to see people and objects in terms of their ability to provide him with supplies. Searching always for his own gratification, he never develops a capacity for giving of himself and never perceives clearly the reality of what the world offers.

With this brief, general description of the oral personality, let us turn now to our own individual case histories for a greater understanding of the orally determined overeater.

HARRY: 800 POUNDS AND DEPRIVED

The first case is one of the most striking examples of an overeater we have encountered. We will call this man Harry. When he came to us, Harry was thirty-four, 6'6", and weighed 800 pounds. Largely because of his immense bulk, his right knee had become unstable. Obviously, no orthopedic surgeon would operate on such a knee until the patient lost weight, to assure some possibility of recovery from surgery. We admitted Harry to a metabolic research floor for a thorough endocrine evaluation and for a program of weight loss. In order merely to provide a room for Harry, special arrangements had to be made on the ward. The patient slept on two beds which were wired together. Since he could not get to the bathroom because the door was too small for him to squeeze through, one side of the cubicle was removed.

Harry had a frighteningly grotesque eating history. Yet when he related his food habits, he did so with a matter-of-fact detachment. He described sitting down to a dozen eggs, or two large pizzas, or two whole chickens, as though he were not even talking about himself. He did not seem to take responsibility for his behavior.

Harry had no mother. Physically, of course, she existed. However, she stopped caring for him shortly after giving birth to him. She did not provide a substitute mother to nurture Harry, but simply abandoned him emotionally. His father eventually deserted the family as well. Harry was the oldest of several brothers and sisters, and he was often asked to help care for the younger children. There was no one to care for him.

If Harry had actually lost his mother, he would most probably have been better able to cope with the desertion. If she had died, for example, he may have been able to live with an idealization of her, a fantasy of how she might have provided for him had she been alive. But instead she *was* there, supplying no provisions for him. Harry remembered returning home to find only his father there waiting for his mother, who frequently never came home. Later, after his father disappeared, he often came home to find his mother sexually involved with various men, ignoring Harry's presence.

Without a mother, the boy received no nurturance, no security, nothing to trust. The world around him provided no alternative sources of physical or emotional caring. His life was to become a continual, desperate search for those much-needed supplies.

In his search he found a lovely young woman who grew up in a home with an abundance of food. His food had usually consisted of the scraps and leftovers from his mother's meals. It was the first time Harry ever realized that so much food existed. His girlfriend's house had three freezers downstairs, two refrigerators upstairs, which was rather bizarre in itself. She herself was thin and did not eat much, though she liked to cook and to feed people. For Harry, she offered all the nurturance he longed for. He wanted her for a mother.

The couple got married. His wife began to cook and Harry began to eat—copiously. Because his wife could never replace his mother, she never could make up to Harry the love he did not get from his mother. For that reason, no matter how much she fed him, his hunger was never satisfied. Sometimes Harry ate six or seven steaks a day. His wife began feeding him all day long.

Harry developed hoarding behavior. He spent more and more time in his bedroom, where he kept large supplies of food, three television sets, and several radios. The mounds of fat that accumulated on his body were another grotesque form of hoarding. It was also a symbolic incorporation of his missing mother. No matter how much he had to eat, he never felt certain that his source of food would be secure, and so he ate for tomorrow and the next day and the next. The hoard he kept in his bedroom made it a symbolic womb, the epitome of a nurturing environment. Even his choice of nonfood items revealed Harry's desire to be passively cared for: the televisions and radios "fed" him information about the outside world, entertained him, and provided companionship.

Let us now try to analyze in greater detail how Harry perceived his world. It should come as no great surprise that the oral personality has difficulty assuming responsibility. The oral stage is the earliest stage of development, during which time the mother or mother substitute *is* the responsible world. In the ensuing anal stage, the child begins to develop its own sense of guilt and responsibility. But because of Harry's frustration at the earliest stage of childhood, he continued to have problems that belong to the oral period. He never ceased seeing the world through the eyes of a helpless, irresponsible child.

Harry was unable to take genuine responsibility for his own actions. He reported how much he ate, but in a detached way—as if he himself were not the subject of his reports. How could he control himself on a diet when he could not even feel responsible for his own eating? He wanted to be treated like a baby. He wanted to diet on a hospital metabolic ward where he could be watched and cared for constantly. At home he insisted that his wife feed him in his womb-like bedroom. He seemed incapable of assuming responsibility for what his wife was doing, and he had enormous difficulty with the responsibilities involved in raising his own children.

Magical thinking was also part of Harry's frightened world. He felt his weight had appeared magically, and so would disappear magically as well. He perceived an unreal quality in his eating behavior and in the rest of his interaction with the outside world. When face to face with elements of reality, he became uneasy, since reality was what he wanted to escape most. The central core of Harry's reality was that his mother had given him barely enough to survive—a perception too painful to acknowledge. To avoid this overwhelming rejection, he had had to devise an unreal world of supplies he could hoard. Harry felt most at ease in a dream-like state, watching the magic of television in his bedroom, shades pulled down, sunglasses on, and being fed continually. (This description brings to mind the drug addict, also a primitive oral personality, most comfortable in a passive dream-like state of drug intoxication.)

Harry's relationships with people, including his wife, were not very real to him because he himself felt unreal. He actualized this unreal quality by creating in himself a size and shape that seemed equally unreal. More a mountain than a man, he was somehow more at ease with this grotesque mass surrounding his body. The very idea of weight loss made him feel anxious.

Harry was a passive person—a typical oral trait. He needed to be given to, cooked for. He had not developed a sense of initiative which would allow him to actively enter into the real world and dare to take chances there. He clung to the comfortable passive state—in bed, watching television, eating.

Harry was also very self-centered—another factor in orality. The term primary narcissism refers to this infantile form of self-centeredness. Harry wanted to receive and receive, always asking for supplies without any real capacity for giving in return. As an infant he had sensed that his survival was tenuous. It seemed frighteningly urgent that he receive enough to stay alive, a feeling so devastating that in adulthood he continued to consider his mere survival an urgent matter. The world he lived in revolved solely around him.

When Harry was given a battery of psychological tests, his primary narcissism and his inability to look at the world objectively became even clearer. For example, when he was asked to interpret a picture of a boy riding a bike, he responded according to his emotions. Instead of saying that he saw a boy riding a bike, he said, "This picture is scary to me." His response was to the affective component of an internal reality, subjective and self-centered.

Infants have a diffuse view of the world and are unable to differentiate themselves from the countless sights, sounds and emotions surrounding them. The mother is a crucial part of this world. The child's mouth is central to its survival and to its pleasure. Merging feelings are centered in its mouth, through which the mother is experienced. The mother and the whole world can thus be "swallowed up" and become part of the child's inner self. In a sense, then, the surrounding world not only envelops the infant, but becomes part of the core of the infant's self.

As the child matures and develops, it learns to separate from other persons and objects in the world. The primitive symbiosis or feeling of oneness with mother and environment begins to dissipate. Areas of the body other than the mouth become increasingly important. The feeling that the world can be taken in through the mouth gradually loses its strength as more sophisticated views of reality develop.

However, for oral personalities such as Harry, these feelings and this world view remain essentially unchanged. As an adult, Harry continued to feel that he could swallow up his world. Since he never truly matured emotionally, he continued to be burdened by what he had incorporated as an infant. He had "swallowed" the weaknesses of his provider—his mother—and made them his own. Her bad feelings were now part of him, giving him very negative feelings about himself. This self-hatred, buried early and deeply within him, was manifest in the destructive quality of his eating behavior. (Again we see the parallel in the self-destructive incorporating behavior of the drug addict: overeating for Harry and injection of intoxicating drugs for the addict permit them to experience merging feelings as well as a sense that the real self is being deservedly punished.)

Harry chose a wife who he felt would help him stay afloat. He hoped that somehow she could become the super-provider. Like other patients we have seen, Harry found an ongoing life situation which allowed him to sustain his emotional struggle. His marriage eventually became yet another part of his illness and represented his infantile solution to his problem. Marriages such as his have difficulty enduring. But when they do, they help perpetuate the problem because the relationship offers a false solution to what is troubling one or both spouses.

Ultimately, Harry became severely disappointed in his wife, since the basic distrust he had of his mother was merely transferred to his wife. Though she cooked for him almost continually, he never trusted that she would present him with a meal the next day. When we asked Harry's wife why she supplied him with so much food, she admitted that she was afraid he would kill her if she did not. She sensed his urgency, his distrust, and his desperation. As the mother substitute, she was the target for all the buried hatred Harry had for his real mother. Harry felt power when he ate, power to consume and destroy. Somehow knowing this, his wife feared for her own destruction. She feared Harry's emotional wish to swallow up, or incorporate, his whole world, of which she was a central part.

Their bizarre relationship has continued for years because, in part, his wife's own problems find some strange solution in it as well. She is a woman who feels unworthy of having her own needs and desires met and seeks to exist primarily as a provider for Harry's needs. The reasons for her pathology are not pertinent here, except in helping us to realize the extent to which the marriage is permeated by a mutual meshing of two devastating problems.

In summary, it must be stated that Harry is our most extreme example of an oral cluster overeater. Prominent in his personality are an inability to tolerate tension, an urgency to eat and to incorporate orally, a lack of basic trust, an inability to give, an inability to accept personal responsibility, magical thinking, an unreal quality to his perceptions of the world, an exaggerated need for nurturance, passivity, narcissism, and a feeling of omnipotence. If many of these traits are present in obese patients, and if they are quite pronounced, the overeaters must be treated as part of the oral cluster. Recognizing this helps the physician or therapist to understand how the overeater views the world and why responsibility for adhering to a diet is so extremely difficult for such a person to assume. Specific treatment for this type of overeater will be discussed in Chapter 10.

DOLLY: THE 25-YEAR-OLD BABY

The case of Dolly is also illustrative of an oral cluster overeater. Dolly, living in a twenty-five-year-old body weighing 300 pounds, looks like an enormous baby. She often sits in a fetal position, swaying her body back and forth. She seems to want to be picked up and rocked, and one might respond to her that way if only she did not weigh so much. She is all roundness: her breasts appear to be part of her abdomen; her cheeks are full; her face is smooth, with no apparent wrinkles.

Dolly's immaturity is revealed in her girlish gestures, attire, and habits. She loves sweets and foods she can suck, sip, lick, or otherwise consume slowly. Her movements too are slow and small, flowing and adapting to her environment—typical characteristics of persons in the oral cluster. Weight loss or signs of aging would probably be very frightening to Dolly. Once her "baby fat" disappeared, she would look more like an adult, but the problem remaining would be that she would not feel like an adult. Her body-image would then be incompatible with her self-image— a terrifying new reality.

Dolly's infantile self-image has its roots in her earliest relationship with her mother. This relationship thwarted her development as an independent person. Dolly did not have a true separate identity, so fused was she with her mother. The symbiosis was so pervasive during the oral stage that Dolly was unable to advance toward maturity later on.

As in Harry's case, Dolly's oral personality stemmed from an abnormal relationship with her mother at the oral stage of development. Whereas Harry was totally frustrated by lack of maternal care at that stage, Dolly had an overly close relationship with her mother. Both experiences were negative, leaving the two unable to progress through a normal childhood. Like Harry, Dolly did not develop feelings of independence, personal responsibility, and initiative.

It was Dolly's mother who created the identity problems between herself and her daughter. The father was a weak man who did not intervene or have much effect on what was happening between mother and daughter. The mother's own problems were manifested in her strong need to live her life through her daughter's existence. Dolly was "used" to act out a part of her mother's neurosis. During the oral stage, Dolly incorporated both her mother's care and her mother's needs—the most prominent of which was the need to fuse her life with her daughter's.

Dolly's mother needed to find some reason for her own day-to-day existence. As soon as her daughter was born, she made caring for the infant her prime purpose and activity. No wonder she had to keep Dolly from growing up: she had no purpose in life otherwise. The message given unconsciously to Dolly was that, other than caring for a baby, there was no meaning or purpose to life. The only value for Dolly's mother, and thus for Dolly, was in retaining an immutable existence between the two.

Since Dolly was unable to develop beyond the oral stage, she, like Harry, was never able to free herself of this very strong maternal need which she had incorporated. Because this was happening during the oral stage, when the mouth was the central mode of experiencing the world, Dolly's need to fuse with her mother became evident in later life through her compulsive eating behavior. For both Harry and Dolly, overeating reflected a basic underlying problem—the problem of fusion. By overeating they hoped to recreate a feeling of oneness with the primitive womb-like world of infancy.

As Dolly became older, her behavior appeared to become more independent, but even her apparent independent behavior was meant to win her mother's approval. During later stages of development, such as toilet training, when she achieved new skills, Dolly never internalized any genuine feelings of accomplishment—underlying her achievements was still the overriding need to do things for her mother. Her accomplishments, opinions, and feelings were not based on her own needs, but rather on the incorporated needs of her mother. Though we all do things to please our mothers even when our mothers are long deceased, for Dolly this was a pervasive way of being that prevented nearly all truly independent action and thought.

Dolly is a low achiever, with no career and no income. People so invested in keeping themselves from ever leaving infancy behind them are usually low achievers. Like Dolly, they rarely lose their tempers; they don't "make waves." Dolly does not like to travel: if she has to take a trip, it is carefully planned to avoid uncertainty. She does not gamble because she does not trust fate. This fundamental lack of trust results in her doing little and risking little. Since life does not seem to offer much, she cannot risk losing anything.

Dolly, and people like her, appear to grow up but continue to relate closely to their mothers. Dolly was actually living with her mother when she became our patient; others choose to live nearby or may be psychologically very involved in the real or fantasized emotional demands of their mothers. Frequently their problem worsens suddenly because they do manage to break away and move, or because their mothers become ill or die before the child has resolved the problem of fusion and separation.

SUMMARY

The case histories of Dolly and Harry are unusual. Many overeaters, as we shall see, have personalities that are far less primitive and many have matured beyond the oral stage. Their personalities usually reflect the problems of later stages of development. However, all people with eating problems have some traits and needs belonging to the oral cluster. Overeaters frequently return to oral gratifications and consolations when coping with problems. They lived through the oral stage, they know their mouths to be a source of satisfaction.

In some sense, therefore, overeating is a mechanism whose goal is fusion with mother, the ultimate provider. Individuals belonging to the oral cluster repeat, over and over again, their need for food, nurturance, and protection. These are the supplies they absolutely needed for survival during the oral stage of development, the first year of life. Because of the serious problems that engulfed them during that year, the themes of the oral stage are echoed throughout their later lives.

4

The Angry Overeater

The Anal Cluster

THE DYNAMICS

*A*ngry and depressed, trying not to let their feelings show, asking for a diet but needing to binge, some overeaters struggle in a personality trap that we call the anal cluster. More patients fit this category than any other. Strangely enough, they are not all fat, they do not all act angry, and often they even manage to cover up their depression. But they will tell a physician or therapist that overeating is a pervasive problem for them. What in their development is responsible for their overeating? What does all this carefully concealed anger, depression, and binging mean?

People who belong to this eating cluster have their primary "weak spots" at the anal stage. They have passed through the oral stage of development with sufficient success. Therefore, in general, they do not have the problems discussed in the last chapter or at least such problems are not primary issues for the rest of their lives. Having basically gained the capacity to accept their environment and to trust their mother at the oral stage, they now enter (at around the age of two) the anal stage centering on toilet training.[1]

When the child learns control of his bowel movements, he learns that the act depends on his initiative alone. He learns that he can produce an effect on his environment—he can make people angry or pleased by his actions.

At the same time, other important signs of independence start emerging. The child now is developing new motor skills. At the oral stage of development he accepted his mother's milk; now he can throw a plate of food on the floor if he does not like it or simply walk away from it. If he is thwarted completely, a genuine sense of independence and initiative does not develop. Clearly, much of a child's independent behavior during the anal stage is involved with anger.

Initiative and anger are closely linked, since the parent must inevitably put some restrictions on the child. If the limits and restrictions are too numerous, the child gets very angry because the expression of his "natural" instincts is being prevented. The child may have to suppress or bury his anger, which in later life may seem all the more powerful because of its unknown origins. This primitive anger will have magical powers attached to it, since it evolved in the irrational mind of a toddler and was then buried.

Therefore, the adult who has basic problems in dealing with his or her independence usually has difficulty expressing anger and usually has very little self-esteem. Their "weak spot" is at the anal stage. Understanding the anal character is crucial in the study of overeating, since we have found this type to be very common in the obese. Although many obese patients have difficulty expressing anger or suffer from a poor sense of self-worth, only those for whom questions of independence are central are considered as belonging to the anal cluster.

The anal stage is a stage of "holding on" and "letting go." It is, of course, the development of muscular maturity that allows a child to control bladder and bowel and to become toilet trained naturally. Control of his body now gives the child a way of controlling the responses of those around him. If he holds on until the appropriate time and place, then lets go, he pleases the people around him. This makes him proud of himself—the beginning of self-esteem. If his efforts here are clearly thwarted, the child can never really develop a sense of trust in his own body and will have trouble expressing a full range of emotions and accepting himself.

Another concept intimately involved in anal issues is the feeling of disgust. The following is an example of how this feeling can develop. The mother gives the child a plate of string beans. The child looks at the beans and dumps them on the floor because they are disgusting to him. The child wants ice cream instead and is angry. His action is an independent one. During the anal stage, therefore, disgust leads to independent and angry behavior— feelings that are all connected in the mind of the toddler. However, the mother sees only the angry behavior and herself angrily picks up the beans and forces the child to eat them. This action tells the child that he cannot express anger; he must eat the food; he should not feel disgust. After regaining her composure, the mother reassures the child that the string beans are delicious, not permitting his feeling of disgust to be validated. Opposition, anger, rebellion, and self-assertiveness are thus regarded as "bad" behavior.

The feeling of disgust develops early. If the child is forced to deny it, then he or she may not be able to truly feel other strong emotions in later life. Inability to feel disgust can become a central issue: the child who once threw string beans on the floor still is disgusted by them but must "swallow" his disgust and develop a new defense. Instead of chewing, savoring, and assimilating the string beans, he gulps them down quickly and nearly whole.

The foundations of body-image are developing at this crucial time. The child hated the string beans and now they are inside his body. The magical and primitive concept of "You are what you eat" is part of the child's ideation. The string beans which were disgusting to him have become part of him. The child feels disgust for himself and his self-esteem is diminished. If such incidents occur often in the child's early life, he will later have difficulty feeling strong emotions such as anger and disgust and will have a low self-esteem. Without the capacity to feel and express strong emotions, the child—and later the adult—feels less than alive. This description aptly characterizes those persons belonging to the anal cluster.

Alienation, another important character trait of the anal cluster, develops from the gulping response. We have described how the child learns to gulp the string beans down quickly as a defense against his feeling of disgust. By not chewing and savoring them, he at least avoids some of the disgust. However, as Fritz Perls writes, this is a costly defense.[2] By not chewing the food, he does not wholly assimilate it. The food goes down "as is." The string beans are not dissolved and transformed by the child, who therefore feels that the food is somewhat foreign to him ("You are what you eat"). At a time when body-image is just developing, the child feels that his body is not really his but also somewhat foreign. Since this alienation occurs at such an early stage of development, it becomes a deep-seated, irrational form of alienation that is hard to deal with.

The separation of the body from the inner self is a primitive alienation. This sense of separateness is basic to the anal cluster. Furthermore, as we shall see when we discuss individual cases, this very alienation from the inner self becomes a basic defense mechanism in dealing with stress. If your body is not really you, then trauma to or criticism of your outer self—the self the world sees—cannot hurt or affect you deeply. The real you is in an inner shell protected by mounds of fat.

Weight reduction for the anal type can be dangerous in that it symbolizes the loss of a basic defense mechanism. The fear of too much weight loss is the fear that the true inner self—full of anger—will be exposed. The obese patient in this cluster frequently reaches a weight plateau and either refuses, consciously or unconsciously, to go below it. Since the anger is so primitive and deep, the great fear is that if it came out it would be very powerful and damaging. Therefore, over-compensatory behavior keeps it in check: this type of patient appears to the outside world as a low-keyed, unaggressive, nice guy. He is living a lie and deep down he knows it. He *must* live the lie, he feels, or he could hurt, and therefore, be hurt. He cannot expose himself by shedding his fat.

It is not surprising that the person has created such a distorted image of what the fat is doing on his body, long after childhood has gone. He needed that protective shell very early in life, when his body-image was first beginning to develop. Since this distortion developed so early, it is extremely difficult to deal with in therapy. It is wholly irrational and basic to the patient's personality.

Experts in child development, among them Erik Erikson, are convinced that a child going through the anal stage needs to live in an environment that has control.[3] As an infant in the oral stage, the child came to feel a basic trust in his world and moved on to the anal stage. There he needs to feel that he will not be jeopardized by the exercise of his own choices in holding on and letting go. Firmness will protect him and give him a feeling of stability while he learns the appropriate and inappropriate ways of letting go. It takes a while for his musculature to gain the ability to always hold on and let go with discretion.

We have found that obese people with alcoholic parents tend to belong to the anal cluster. Control and the avoidance of anger are very important issues for them. The alcoholic parents, who created the young child's environment, did not always provide an orderly world. The child often was exposed to violent displays of rage that appeared meaningless and arbitrary. (Alcohol is known to lower inhibitions against anger.) These disruptive explosions are devastating to the young child who needs to develop self-control and self-esteem. The child would have liked—in fact needed—to depend on his parents to maintain control for him while he was trying to master the ability himself. His disappointment, shame, and doubt in experiences where control is lost may affect him much later in life.

We have seen patients who are terribly afraid that they will lose control of their feelings. These men and women, who fall into the anal cluster, cannot risk strong emotions, especially anger. They fear that if they were to let go of their anger, it might be uncontrolled. One woman whose mother was an alcoholic told her therapist she would like to get angry but decided against it because she was certain her rage would be destructive and she might easily tear down the stone walls in the therapist's office. A man in a dance-oriented form of therapy said that he had better not use the therapist's drum because he would surely hit it so hard as to break it.

The anal cluster is characterized by compulsive behavior centering around the issue of control. When persons of this type feel out of control, they will—instead of having temper tantrums that they fear will destroy the things around them—turn the anger in on themselves, stuffing food into themselves indiscriminately. They strengthen their external shell of fat, while simultaneously "stuffing" their feelings.

The woman who did not tear down her therapist's stone wall left her session and bought food, eating compulsively in her automobile. She sensed that this activity was truly dangerous to her safety, and she was in fact risking the destruction of her car and herself by eating while driving. She knew, as other overeaters know, that such behavior was bad. (Overeating is often indulged in simply because it *is* bad.) She exposed her primitive inner self, a self that had much concealed anger. She behaved badly and therefore felt she must be punished. At her next session she reported what she had done to the therapist. He gave her a physical activity to perform as a means of ventilating her anger. Keeping in mind her own fantasies of tearing down his wall, he asked her if she would be able to tear an entire telephone book given the strength of her fantasized rage. She fantasized that she could do this, too. He brought her the book and she quickly discovered that she could not rip it up. Then the therapist gave her permission to rip pages out until she felt better. She tore the entire book, pulling apart a few pages at a time. She then looked around her, apologized for the mess, and said she would clean it up. The therapist reassured her that it was not a mess, that she had in fact done nothing to be ashamed of, nothing for which she should be punished.

The man who was afraid to use his therapist's drum had many sessions in which he joked about what he would do to that drum if he ever got hold of it. Actually, it was always available to him although he feared handling it and the anger associated with it. Finally, he did pick it up and the sounds he made were violently loud. But the drum did not break. He giggled, shedding his tension through laughter. He beat the drum and giggled some more. After many sessions he began to use the drum as an instrument of control. He and his therapist agreed that she would move to any rhythm he beat. By controlling how fast or how slow she moved and when she stopped or started he was able to gain confidence in his own power and ability to assert himself in a non-destructive way.

These patients were afraid to risk being angry for fear of losing control of their feelings. They had not been permitted to acquire this ability in their formative years and so had to experiment, test, and create control mechanisms as adults. The food they gorged on served to push down the anger, to control explosive feelings by burying the affect under the food. (Physically, large quantities of food act as a depressant, slowing down bodily movements and blunting initiative and feelings.) But because loss of control is always a dangerous and ever-present possibility, they tended to allow themselves to lose control only in one way —with food. By eating compulsively, they were assured that the damage and destruction would be unleashed more upon themselves than upon anyone else.

For the anal person food serves another important purpose. Overeating creates a weight problem, which results in a new activity: dieting. The diet becomes of supreme importance. It is the ultimate symbol of control. Disgust is repressed; anger is repressed; emotions are repressed. The dieter feels good about himself and spends much time discussing his food intake with other overweight people— witness the proliferation of weight-watching clubs and groups in our society. The dieter is also willing to pay a doctor a rather large fee in order to maintain his diet. These compulsive dieters are not simply interested in losing weight; it is important that their doctor, and all persons involved in their treatment, be aware of what emotional significance the diet has to them. Others enter into the dieter's pathology when they focus on the diet, since above all else the patient wants control and wants to avoid strong feelings. If the dieter starts feeling anger—or any other overwhelming feelings—he may go on a binge.

Binging becomes linked to strong feelings. This type of person eats when agitated or nervous. If he goes to the refrigerator nearly every time he feels strong anger, eventually the refrigerator itself begins to represent anger. A diet, therefore, can mean the denial of emotional life. A binge can represent emotional turbulence. Early in life the anal cluster patient learned that emotions are dangerous, bad, and difficult to control. The childhood response was to suppress the feeling. Now, as an adult, a food binge means that emotional life has erupted again and that control has been lost. Dieting allows the person to regain self-esteem through reinstating control.

Food represents contradictory things to the anal type: it can be linked favorably to strong feelings and can suppress such feelings; it can be used as a form of self-punishment or as a reward. Cycles of binging and dieting reflect the anal patient's ambivalent attitude toward food and the act of eating.

Difficulties during the anal stage of development can produce anxiety about being independent and being on one's own. Instead of ever really becoming independent, or when independent behavior is required of them, people in the anal cluster are likely to eat. The eating takes them back to the nurturing oral stage, when they could exist in symbiotic closeness with the adult who cared for them. The extra food and weight they acquire may symbolize that symbiosis: the food is the other person they were so dependent on, and by eating it they incorporate that important person. In his mind, therefore, the overweight person never really has to develop autonomy, for he "carries" the other person around with him in the form of excess fat.

Separation from family, friends, or familiar settings and routines can cause anxiety later in life for people who had trouble in initially establishing independent controls. The anxiety is often accompanied by self-doubt and a lack of self-confidence. The return to nurturing, eating behavior is an attempt to fill the void created by separation and to mitigate the fear of being alone.

For all these reasons it is obvious why the obese person in the anal cluster has so much difficulty maintaining weight loss after dieting. As we have stated, binging can be an expression of strong feelings or a form of self-punishment. If the patient diets and simply loses weight but still has a need to suppress feelings, especially anger, then he will eventually and inevitably have a need to punish himself for feeling that anger. This will in turn reawaken the need to binge and the patient will regain his weight.

Thus it will be virtually impossible for him to set a pattern of reasonable food intake on a daily basis.

The reader may now wonder, "I'm not very fat, but I have many other characteristics of the obese group just described. I am either always dieting or overeating, but I am able to maintain a reasonable weight by dieting much of the time. I too have fears of being independent. I have trouble with strong feelings, especially anger. Do I fit into the anal cluster?"

Even though such a reader is not obese or seriously overweight, we would say he does have an eating problem associated with the anal cluster. This cluster best describes the basic aspects of his personality, and while other issues may be involved in his eating problem, anal issues are central.

As it happens, overeating does not always result in obesity. Sometimes the result is a "stocky" or "pleasantly plump" figure or simply a few extra pounds, which can be disguised with a clever wardrobe. But if eating is compulsive, with an alternating pattern of binges and dieting, there is clearly an emotional hunger operating. No diet will result in permanent weight loss or even in consistent maintenance of weight so long as the emotions remain buried or unexpressed.

Depression is another characteristic of the anal cluster that we must consider at this point. Many patients in this cluster have a tendency to be depressed. Their inability to feel or to tolerate strong emotions is part of the sense of emptiness often seen in depressed persons. Self-punishment is another aspect of depression. Otto Fenichel has emphasized that a loss of self-esteem usually precipitates a depression, and patients in the anal cluster are usually struggling with low self-esteem. Lack of initiative, lack of energy, sluggishness, or immobility may also be present. In the extreme, one sees a near total paralysis—a sign of deep depression.

What happens to eating behavior when people become

depressed? Most people tend to decrease their food intake or even to refuse food altogether if the depression is severe enough. Eating, after all, requires action and depression is marked by an inability to act. Food is seen by most as a reward, but when self-esteem is low many people are unable to allow themselves that reward.

People in the anal cluster typically display a very different eating behavior when they are depressed. They may gorge themselves with food—their own peculiar form of self-punishment. If, for example, the overeater is angry at someone but feels he cannot express or even acknowledge his anger, he punishes himself instead by "stuffing" himself and suppressing the emotion. He knows his overeating will cause an accumulation of fat—a detested punishment.

Since depression is linked to self-hate, one response to it is self-punishment. For an anal cluster person experiencing self-loathing, overeating is both the symbol of and the punishment for his feelings of inadequacy. Though overeating always requires an action, in anal types it is a compulsive, sometimes almost unconscious action. Therefore it never shows true initiative.

During an acute depression, feelings of hopelessness can become overwhelming. Chances of living without strong feelings seem more difficult than ever at such times. For the anal cluster person, self-control often disappears with the onset of depression. If he has been dieting successfully until then, he will probably be unable to maintain the control necessary to remain on the diet. Overeating will follow, as the thought of growing slim becomes ever more remote and hopeless. The physician should consider medical treatment of an underlying depression in such cases. Antidepressant medication may help curb appetite or the compulsive urge to eat. If the patient does have an underlying depression—frequently quite difficult to detect—a trial of antidepressants may be extremely helpful. It is this chronic depression that can provoke compulsive binging. Whenever something happens to undermine their precariously low self-esteem, anal cluster patients may gorge themselves.

ELLEN: THE COCL, CALM, AND COLLECTED BINGE EATER

This is the story of Ellen. Ellen is a gainer and a loser, always either dieting or binging. To the outer world she maintains an attractive appearance and speaks in a voice that is always soft and modulated. Most significantly, she consistently maintains a calm, controlled manner. When she feels upset, it is a cold feeling, never hot. There are no temper tantrums or loud battles in her life. Yet when Ellen is anxious or depressed, she eats—for days on end, continuously, keeping her activities to a minimum, making certain that food is involved in as many of her activities as possible. When she is feeling better and is able to increase her activities again, she breaks the cycle of overeating and diets strenuously to try to lose the weight she has gained.

Ellen's history reveals the importance of the issue of independence in anal cluster persons. She was an only child, born after her mother had suffered four miscarriages. Very much wanted and awaited, she became the sole love object for her parents and assumed the burden of being all their lost children to them. In this atmosphere of smothering love and overprotection, she was unable to evolve her true self. Self-actualization for her as an adult is still related to the primitive internalization of her parents.

What we see today in Ellen is a very refined, poised, and well-dressed young woman. When she seeks professional help for her weight problem, she is given a diet. But because her inner self has continued to exist primarily on the emotional level that was so crucial to her parents she needs something else. Her way of internalizing her parents is still the way of a young child—sucking and eating. Instead of actualizing her true independent self, she actualizes a version of her self that is aimed at maintaining her connection to her mother and father.

Ellen can never really internalize her parents by eating —none of us can. And that is why her behavior is repetitive and compulsive. It is doomed never to be successful. Though her parents are alive and healthy, she lives with tremendous fear of their death. In fact, she has never strayed far from them; her home is close to her parents'. Her husband works for her father. Because she is so unsure of her own inner individuality, she fears that when her parents die she will lose her externalized self.

When we look at a person's psychological development in this way, we begin to see what role eating plays in their emotional life. For Ellen it served the function of reassuring her of her own existence at a stressful period in her life. The food was real; therefore she was real, she existed, she was alive. The need for external and concrete proof of her existence relates to her childhood problem of feeling like a person only in terms of two people outside herself— her parents. Ellen never grew up enough to feel her separate existence from that of her mother and father.

Ellen's body-image reflected this problem as well. She felt she was "fatter" than she actually was. Her psychological identity was tenuous and her sense of her physical boundaries was equally unstable. She was never quite sure where her parents stopped and she began. When she ate, she was in a sense incorporating her parents, making herself bigger, so that she could contain both of them. Another reason for "fattening up" was that there had to be enough of her to fill the needs of everyone close to her—her children, her husband, her mother, and her father.

Ellen has many characteristics in common with obese people in the oral cluster, especially with respect to boundary and separation problems. After studying her overall personality, however, we diagnosed her problems as lying mainly in the anal cluster. Unlike oral patients such as Harry and Dolly, Ellen was able to receive strength during her oral stage of development. She developed a strong sense of trust in her parents. Ironically, this trust was so strong that it affected her ability to resolve the crucial problems that arise at the later anal stage. She had trouble leaving the security of the oral stage and was very reluctant to move on in her development.

Unfortunately, Ellen is unable to recollect specific events that may have occurred during the anal stage of her life. We can hypothesize from what we know of her parents, their needs, and the family dilemma at that time what some of those events might have been. We will turn to the hypothetical example of the string beans to see what might have happened to Ellen when she first entered the stage of independent choices, personal initiative, and disgust.

Let us say that baby Ellen's mother offers her string beans for dinner one night. The smell and taste of the beans fills Ellen with disgust. But she completely trusts her mother, since everything else her mother has given her until this time has been good. She trusts that the string beans must be good too, and she eats them calmly. (In this respect Ellen differs from most anal overeaters, who eat hastily.) Without rebelling, without throwing the food away or gulping it down, she does what is expected of her.

Later in life, we know that Ellen does the same thing. She quickly learns what is expected of a person in her social class and situation and does it. Conformity and approval from parental authority figures are her prime values. As she matures, she realizes with frightening impact that she is *always* doing what her parents and the rest of the world want her to do, and never what she herself independently desires. She has carefully "chewed" and "swallowed" what her parents gave her. She has internalized them so well that she is now a mirror-image of them; she has lost her true self.

Ellen has not been permitted to learn how to achieve independence. She does not have in her repertoire of behavior the acts of spitting out or rejecting what is given her. Since she never really experienced the rudimentary beginnings of independent action, she does not know what she wants separate from what her parents want. Consequently, she cannot really rebel. She does what is expected of her . . . she eats the detested string beans and thinks she likes them. A dangerous split ensues between her gut reactions and her intellectual responses—a split of which she is not even consciously aware.

Like the typical patient in the anal cluster, Ellen is alienated from her own feelings. These feelings are so amorphous and poorly developed in the first place, however, that there can be no real fight for their expression. There can be no real choice. When she is upset, she does not feel the deeper, genuine anger. Intellectually, she knows that she should, and so once again she does what is expected of her and makes the "proper" choice or response. But her gut feelings are not there. She senses that as an adult woman she *should* be feeling anger in the gut, but she cannot bring it into consciousness. Nevertheless, and typically, she trusts that "everything will all work out in the end."

Ellen trusts the world, as she trusted her parents. For her, overeating is an affirmation of this trust. She trusted her mother and so ate the string beans—symbols of that trust. When, as an adult, she had to deal with reality and discovered that, unfortunately, everything does not work out, she allayed her anxiety and angry disappointment by overeating, again and again. While she ate, calmness and tranquility reigned. At those moments she could trust that her problems would somehow be solved. This repetitive behavior helped her avoid spontaneous, independent action and strong feelings, both of which presented her with enormous difficulty.

Intellectually, Ellen was intelligent enough to realize that life is not "a bowl of cherries." She even realized that everything probably would *not* work out. She understood the futility of her child-like, neurotic pattern of overeating and wanted to face issues that she knew needed to be confronted, since "growing up" was also expected of her. Overeating is her infantile weakness, the escape she allows herself from doing what is expected.

Having decided that she wanted to diet effectively, Ellen consulted us. Her ambivalence about food was the first issue to deal with. Overeating, though symbolic of her child-like acceptance of the world, could not solve her problems as an adult. In treatment she benefited from working in groups where dance and movement were used as part of therapy.

In many ways, Ellen is very atypical of anal overeaters. She did not progress to feelings of independence and had no real initiative. Most others who belong to the anal cluster have at least progressed to the point where they have tested some independent action; they have discovered the possibility of self-assertion and angry behavior. Perhaps as toddlers they tried this kind of behavior but were thwarted in their early efforts. Nevertheless, the anger and initiative remained deep down in their psyches. Being out of touch with these feelings as adults, they perceived their lost emotions as very powerful and irrational whenever they surfaced. Unlike Ellen, these members had the strength to rebel against their parents at the anal stage. As adults, however, they are afraid to do so. They may appear quite passive, while deep down they retain all of their pent-up anger. Since their feelings toward their parents are more strongly ambivalent, many do not accept the world as willingly as Ellen.

MARTIN: THE ALIENATED OVEREATER

This is the story of Martin. He belongs to the anal cluster and is more typical of that group than Ellen. Martin's early childhood history is also typical of anal cluster overeaters: he had one very domineering, cold, rigid parent and one who offered a bit more comfort and warmth but who was too weak to counteract the other's rigidity.

Martin's father was an aloof yet demanding man. If Martin did not live up to his father's expectations, he was verbally degraded. Since Martin's father was a devout Christian Scientist, a central expectation was that Martin would rise above the world of physical pain and illness. He was instructed that his body was not truly real. If he felt pain, his father told him, it was in his mind. He was told to use his mind to control his feelings—reality was supposed to exist entirely in his rational mind and as far as his father was concerned, strong emotions were not part of the rational mind. Martin was forced to deny his feelings, both emotional and physical, in order to gain his father's approval.

One of Martin's early memories is of his father washing off a wound the boy suffered and then saying that "it doesn't really hurt." During these formative years he chastized Martin for not being strong and for "listening" to his feelings. Hence, Martin developed a low self-esteem, particularly regarding his bodily feelings.

In contrast, Martin's mother was warm, but ineffectual. She was a passive woman who allowed her husband to impose his harsh religious and childrearing beliefs upon her without questioning them. She became a rigid feeder: Martin had to eat at particular times, and he had to eat what was given to him. During infancy, if he cried between his feedings, she treated these cries as unreal signals from the baby's body.

Since this attitude was more her husband's than her own, Martin's mother had mixed feelings about what she was doing, and her ambivalence was sensed by Martin. She overcompensated for these cold childrearing practices by being warm and overly protective in other ways, frequently spending a great deal of time with him. Martin recalls that she was "always there."

In this environment Martin's feelings of independence could not develop adequately. He was getting messages from both parents that fostered a low self-esteem: his father contradicted and rejected his bodily needs; his mother was hesitant ever to leave him on his own. Thus the boy had no opportunity to develop a solid sense of independence or to assert his own needs.

Because his authoritarian father would tolerate no disobedience and no expression of emotions, Martin grew up with the sense that his feelings, his body, and especially his anger all had a mysterious strength and power. His mother seemed to show both fear of and a fascination with these traits. By perceiving her strong attraction to and repulsion by anger, Martin not only "tasted" anger—unlike Ellen—but came to believe that his own anger if ever unleashed would be dangerously destructive.

As we have already stated, anal problems center around issues of anger, self-esteem, independence, and alienation —all of which were central issues for Martin. He was unable to trust his own feelings, even his own pain, and soon separated his rational mind from his body and emotions.

What do these anal traits have to do with Martin's eating habits and weight problem? These personality characteristics appear with early eating behavior, with the early choices and decisions of the child. In that behavior are the roots of initiative, and even rebellion. The rigidity of Martin's parents prevented his development of independence. The feeding patterns they imposed forced him to "swallow" his own inclinations, alienating him from his body and damaging his self-esteem. When an overweight Martin was referred to us at the age of thirty-five, he had already been in medical treatment for three years for lower back pain with radiation down both legs. His orthopedic surgeon sent him to us in the hope that Martin could lose some weight to take pressure off his back.

On examination, Martin appeared to be experiencing moderate pain. Otherwise, he seemed rather flat emotionally. He was intelligent and very well-read. In short, his rational mind was highly developed, but his ability to express emotion was lacking. On the surface, he was what his father had always wanted him to be—he had never truly rebelled.

Martin's only apparent "failure" was in complaining of lower back pain. Inevitably, this pain worsened whenever he visited his parents, and was forced to ask his doctor for a narcotic prescription to kill the pain. It is intriguing to speculate here on the psychological meaning in Martin's exacerbated back pain. Merely revealing his back ailments to his father could be seen as a type of rebellion: "Look, Dad! I don't fit the mold you made for me ... I'm having pain ... your religion is a pack of lies ... my pain *does* exist!" But Martin could not rebel openly, could not express anger directly. His only outlet was to express it neurotically and perversely. Indeed, medical doctors had difficulty finding the organic cause of his ailment. Authorities in the field of psychosomatic medicine have documented similar phenomena involving "low back losers," in whom the pain is actually a symptom of psychological pain—and of considerable anger.

When Martin began treatment with us he weighed 250 lbs. He had gained twenty pounds the year before, after his marriage fell apart. His eating habits were not unusual for an anal cluster overeater: he gulped his food down rapidly and overate particularly during times of stress—times when he feared losing control and becoming irrationally angry. His binging at those times was his way of attempting to control and suppress his anger. It also, however, served as an escape from genuinely independent action.

How is binging—which appears to be such an out-of-control type of behavior—a type of control? When Martin's existence was first centered around the crucial issue of control of his body, bowels, and environment, during the anal stage of development, he was faced with a rigid feeder. What and when he ate were directed by his mother.

Self-control was impossible to learn in this area, and was further subverted by an uncompromising father. Later in life, when Martin felt threatened by a loss of self-control due to severe stress (his divorce, for example), he reverted to the eating behavior that allowed him to survive when he was young: he gupled down food, as he had done following his first confrontation with his mother over control of the feeding situation. Binging became hiw form of preventing total self-dissolution. Since the mere desire to binge already made him feel out of control, the act of binging itself gave Martin some semblance of a defense against the crumbling world. It became a controlling defense, one aimed at shoring up his weakened self-esteem.

Binging also allowed Martin to suppress his anger at his parents, who forbade its expressions. By gulping down the foods his mother gave him, he was able to hide his anger from her and later from himself. The food was unwanted —junk. In adulthood he became addicted to "junk food" in order to suppress the same smoldering anger from himself.

Martin was ultimately able to stop binging and start dieting when his anger was at a minimum and his self-esteem fortified. At such times he felt strong enough to deal with stress in healthier ways. He was more accepting of his feelings (negative ones especially) and less alienated from his emotions. At last he could take the long overdue step of rejecting parental feeding. He rejected his father's preconceived notion of what he should be. Diet was now his symbolic refusal to "swallow" what his parents forced him to accept, representing his new sense of independence and self-assertion. During this time Martin also became ready for psychotherapy, trying to analyze and deal with his problems, while continuing to diet.

We have discussed Martin's case in some detail because we feel it demonstrates many of the typical characteristics of the anal cluster overeater, especially with regard to alienation. The child must eat food he does not want or like. If this happens consistently in childhood, it may result in an overall alienation from feelings. Martin's alienation became more marked than usual because of his family's insistence on the teachings of Christian Science —a religion which preaches that bodily pain must be borne without medical intervention.

A Letter from Marie

At this point, we should have some understanding of the anal cluster overeater. The reason for their personality conflicts and their binge eating should be more understandable. The reader may now find it both challenging and illuminating to read a letter from a patient to her doctor describing her very own eating problems and conflicts. Marie, who wrote this letter, is twenty-five years old and is basically an anal cluster overeater. Her letter speaks for itself.

3:15 A.M.
July 23, 1977

Dear Dr. Wise:

Not being able to sleep, I decided to get up and write a few thoughts down. I have trouble expressing myself to you. It is easier to do it this way.

No one has ever asked me the questions you have and I feel really self-conscious talking about myself. As I told you before, I realized that losing weight meant that I would finally have to deal with a few things that I had been avoiding for a long time, consciously or otherwise. Intellectually, I fully understand the whole situation but it's the feelings that get in the way sometimes.

I don't want to make a big deal of this but the fact is I know my father has really had an effect on me. I guess I have been aware of this for a very long time. But the realization has come to me that maybe this is a bigger deal than I have been willing to face up to.

My father is a reserved, quiet person who was very strict with my sister and brother and me while we were growing up. He was distant from us, difficult to talk to, and he believed that children should be seen and not heard. We all learned to live with that. My mother was the exact opposite of my father— warm, loving, and very outgoing. The three of us have always been close to her.

My relationship with my father was one of fear. Of the three of us, I was always the one who never rocked the boat. In spite of his ways, I always loved him and I still do. Lately he has been ok except when he's drinking. Then he gets very argumentative. Underneath he's really a sensitive person but it is a side he doesn't show to many people.

The point of this whole situation is that I have grown up feeling very insecure about men. I never really learned to communicate with them—consequently, with most of the men I met in my life I have formed a protective shield about myself. The minute I thought anyone was seriously interested in me, I chose to flee. I really hate to admit that to you, but I guess I have to.

I really believed that once I lost all of that weight everything would be ok—really ok.

Here I was, really enjoying myself, and I met a guy at a party. We went out for two months. He was a nice guy. It's really hard to meet someone nice, but then when I did, I blew it. Naturally it was my fault. I decided he was making me nervous, and I didn't want to go out with him anymore. I must have given that impression, and I never heard from him again.

At about the same time that happened, I had trouble at work. My new supervisor turned out to make things frustrating for me. My roommate and my family all encouraged me to try a new job, but it was out of town and I really did not want to do it. Finally I went because I thought it would be good for me.

And then my father and I had one of the few blow-outs of all time on Father's Day. With all the above situations, life was a bummer and I got depressed.

Anyway, that's the story. I sent this to you because I didn't want to sit there while you read it.
See you. Thanks,

Marie

Marie is a skillful nurse functioning at a high level in a coronary care unit. In an effort to overcome her self-doubts, she was driven to achieve in her career. Many of the traits attributable to the anal cluster have real value in our society. A well-ordered mind and well-planned goals can be the hallmarks of success.

Olga: The Depressed Pianist with an Alcoholic Mother

Anal qualities of orderliness and controlled emotion, while valued in our society, can be harmful when they prevent a fuller development of the individual. One of our patients, Olga, clearly illustrates the potentially positive aspects of an anal cluster type. The child of an alcoholic mother with an explosive temper, Olga identified with this parent and felt that if she were to express her own anger it too would be "like a volcano."

Olga learned in childhood not to express feelings directly. Instead she used the piano: when she was very angry, she banged on the keys, playing for hours on end. Piano playing became a compulsion—the child's way of dealing with her feelings. Ultimately, her compulsion became an asset, as so often happens in the case of artists. She channeled her anger and her musical talent through rigorous training and became a concert pianist.

Unfortunately, Olga's compulsive behavior also entered into her eating habits. Weight became a physical handicap when she reached the 290-pound mark. She entered treatment for obesity with an underlying depression. Her diet worked well, based on a compulsive system of calorie counting (she was allowed 600 calories a day). Her meals were rigidly structured, which gave her a feeling of control that suited her personality.

In addition to this diet, Olga began antidepressant medication. With it, her self-esteem improved and she was able to accept her feelings and emotions more readily. Instead of burying her feelings with food, she began to examine what she was feeling. One of the things she learned about herself in this way was how intensely she disliked her alcoholic mother—a prime factor in creating dislike for herself.

The real challenge for Olga will begin when she tries to maintain her weight loss without such a rigid diet and without antidepressants. Hopefully, insights and emotional changes that occurred under the influence of psychotherapy will have been enough to change her compulsive eating behavior. A physician cannot call an end to a diet and expect a patient to maintain a reduced weight if the patient has not had some ongoing help with his or her emotional difficulties beforehand.

JACK: THE ANGRY JOGGER WITH AN ALCOHOLIC FATHER

Hidden anger, exertion of will, and independence all appear in the following case study. It is the history of a young obese male whose development was characterized by the continual presence of an alcoholic father from the time of his infancy.

As Jack grew up, he was subjected to repeated scenes of his father's rampages. What Jack saw disgusted him, but being much too young and dependent to do anything about his father's compulsive behavior, he had to accept it, live with it—"swallow it," like the disgusting string beans or whatever other unappetizing food a parent may offer a child. He soon learned this parental lesson: the way to handle anxiety is to put something in your mouth.

During his boyhood and early youth, Jack found that his ambivalence about his father could be acted out in combat sports. He became an extremely tough football player, and throughout his school years ventilated his frustration and anger at his father in this way. He felt disgust not only for the ugly scenes he had been forced to witness, but also for the fruitless efforts his father appeared to make to control his alcoholism.

As Jack grew older, he became absorbed in his career and gave up football. He attempted to keep all strong feelings repressed, especially angry ones. His personal relationships were controlled, and he carefully avoided confrontations involving aggressive, angry feelings. But he began to gain weight as he compulsively overate. Just as his father had used compulsive drinking to deal with the difficulties of adult life, so Jack was now compulsively eating.

In an effort to counteract some of the weight gain, Jack began jogging. This, too, quickly became a compulsion for him. Because of it, he was fortunate enough to be able to stay in good physical condition. Emotionally, however, his needs were not being satisfied by this new sport interest. Compulsive behavior is by its very nature a false solution to emotional problems. It is for this reason a compulsion is repeated over and over again—it never works and must always be attempted again.

Through overeating Jack was trying to control his anger. He felt anger to be a dangerous and overpowering force, since his chief experience with that emotion had been the sight of his father completely enraged and out of control when he was drunk. Combat sports had earlier given him a way of acting out his own anger at his father, but jogging did not release his repressed urge to fight. Jack found himself eating compulsively in order to further repress the anger. But it was there, perilously close to the surface, and he could not run away from the feeling any longer.

Alarmed and upset now not only by his weight gain, but by his inability to control his compulsive eating, Jack sought treatment. In psychotherapy he began to deal with the issue of his anger at his father. Only then was he able to lose weight. The dark, frightening feeling of hating the father he also loved and depended upon as a child was examined in the light of a supportive therapeutic setting. Jack began to understand why he was overeating and to substitute for that self-destructive pattern of behavior the verbal expression of his angry feelings in the comforting presence of his therapist.

The fluctuations in Jack's weight were an important factor in his treatment. Significantly, he regained weight after entering a relationship with a woman he loved. Although the love was mutual and the intimacy generally satisfying, Jack began to re-experience the ambivalence of depending upon a loved one in a close relationship. He again repressed his anxieties and frustrations for fear of jeopardizing the relationship. Unconsciously, he was remembering the anger, disgust, and disappointment caused by his earlier dependency on his father. By holding back these feelings and failing to examine their origin, he resorted to the defense of overeating to cope with his emotions.

Jack's day-to-day relationship with his girlfriend was suffering because he kept avoiding one important part of intimacy—fighting. Not surprisingly, he had no idea of how to fight constructively. His father—a mild, passive, sad person—was not able to express anger unless he was drunk. Jack never saw him get angry in a controlled, adult manner. As most boys do, he identified with his father, and so psychologically acquiesced to that model and to the belief that there is no acceptable way to be angry.

Jack and his girlfriend began a new form of therapy designed to teach couples how to argue fairly. Their relationship became more balanced and healthy, and Jack himself became more alive. The repressed part of his personality was finally able to reveal itself, making it possible for him to put his total self into his love affair for the first time.

We say that people who compulsively overeat when faced with emotional problems are "acting out" their needs primarily in terms of food. Jack was one of these people. It would seem that those forms of psychotherapy that offer direct ways of acting out feelings—psychodrama, bioenergetics, primal therapy—are best for such individuals. These people, like Jack, were never able to use fantasy life or conceptual mental processes to handle their emotional problems well enough. For example, when angry it would never satisfy them merely to conjure up a gruesome mental image of getting revenge on someone—they need to take action. In the case of overeating, the action is turned in upon themselves, until the pain of gorging their bodies stops them.

Jack chose to continue his ongoing exploration of himself through psychodrama, which permits him to act out his emotional life in this way rather than through inappropriate eating behavior. While he is not always happy— many of the feelings he has to deal with and act upon are painful to him—his weight is under control at last because he is not using food to push these feelings back down inside himself. He is discovering healthier outlets for his emotions that his own unhappy father had never been able to teach him.

SUMMARY

As we have seen, food can mean many things to the obese person who fits into the anal cluster. It can serve to strengthen his protective outer shell so that his inner self remains hidden. When strong emotions threaten to erupt, he tends to eat, suppressing his feelings—sometimes doing this so effectively that he does not even *feel* strong feelings as time goes by. Thus, food can become a symbol of non-feeling. Food is compulsively sought when feelings well up. Any strong feeling, good or bad, is dangerous and must be eradicated.

Food also can represent punishment, as we have seen when we discussed the woman who ate and drove her car at the same time, or the disgusted two-year-old forced to swallow string beans in large gulps. We must emphasize and re-emphasize the self-destructive quality of this behavior. As an adult, the patient knows overeating is bad—bad for both medical and cosmetic reasons. Yet the patient compulsively punishes himself for feeling, especially for feeling anger. Mother is no longer there to shove string beans into his mouth; therefore the patient becomes his own "bad" mother by repeating her behavior. This act is a primitive and compulsive act.

For the anal cluster overeater mere dieting is a hopeless solution, since the compulsive, controlling aspects of dieting are just another form of his anal pathology and defense system. For long-term results, issues such as depression, anger, and alienation must be treated, along with the crucial questions of self-esteem and independence. A little simple ventilation of such issues or a great deal of intense, ongoing therapy may be required so that the person may grow emotionally beyond those early childhood problems that are rooted in the anal stage of character development.

5

The Sexual Overeater

The Genital Cluster

THE DYNAMICS

In the treatment of our patients we have been impressed with the frequency of eating problems among people who also have sexual problems. Their troubles arise when they have to deal with their sexuality. This group, which we term the genital cluster, is not easy to treat. In addition to diet, the techniques of psychotherapy must be introduced. Without both, these patients seem to have great difficulty maintaining a lower, more ideal weight.

Overeating as a reaction to problems of sexual identity is apparently more common in women than in men. Excessive eating, taking in "dirty" food—the forbidden fruit—seems to have more sexual implications for women.[1] A man who has trouble with his sexuality or masculinity often strikes out in destructive behavior, which is rarely turned inward. He can also displace his pent-up sexual energies in socially sanctioned areas of aggression and competition—the sports fanatic or workaholic businessman are frequently such types.

The development of a mature sexuality requires that an individual pass comfortably through the genital stage of development.[2] The prior stages of development have certain sexual components, but the genital is the first stage in which sexual differentiation occurs. In it issues of masculinity and femininity are of paramount importance.

The small child has a kind of undifferentiated sexuality that allows him to get excitation and pleasure from many parts of his body. Every kind of activity of which his muscles and his mind are capable (including feelings of pain) can be considered a part of that sexuality. As the child leaves the oral and anal stages—the so-called pregenital stages of development—and achieves genitality, sexual excitement finally becomes centered around the genitals.

An adult whose development is arrested at the pregenital stage is not able to achieve the complete relaxation of a genital climax. Full satisfaction affords the personality many advantages. Physically, regulation of the sex drive is possible, since the person no longer has to dam up the sexual instincts. Instead of living with ambivalent or repressed emotions, the person who has attained genitality is able to fully experience the positive feeling of love and to separate it from negative feelings. This fortunate person is also able to discharge large amounts of sexual excitement directly and at once in a single act: genital orgasm. Such a person does not have the left-over, partial energy that needs to find substitute expressions if it is not to end in neurosis.

The development of this mature form of sexuality is accomplished by satisfactory resolution of genital stage problems. One central issue at this stage of development is resolution of the conflict with the parent of the same sex over possession of the parent of the opposite sex. The little girl, for example, wants Daddy's attention and is jealous of her mother's relationship with him. One way she can resolve her problem is to identify with her mother.[3] Of course the little boy also resolves his guilt over desiring his mother by identifying with his father.

A girl's positive identification with her mother is part of developing genital sexuality. She strives to achieve this by dressing up in Mommy's clothes, even perhaps imitating her speech, gestures, temper, and attitudes. Through such play she is learning to be a woman, especially a woman like her mother—for then her father will wish to "marry" her. Most girls eventually identify with their mothers so well that when they are grown they frequently find themselves involuntarily interacting with their own children in some of the same negative ways their mothers dealt with them and cannot easily free themselves of these less desirable maternal introjects.

Now let us look at some of the possible pitfalls in the development of the young girl's sexuality and femininity. Perhaps her mother is not good at getting her father's love and attention. Or maybe she is not someone the little girl really likes—perhaps there is even something about her mother that the little girl despises. We have treated many patients with weight problems who have had severe difficulties in precisely this area. This has been true to such an extent, in fact, that we feel the subject of sexual identity must be investigated in all patients with persistent weight problems.

RENA: BEING A WOMAN AND FEELING DIRTY

The case of Rena typifies many of the distortions of femininity that may exist in overeaters belonging to the genital cluster. Her story is one of extreme and difficult early childhood conflicts.

Rena's mother was an alcoholic, so absorbed in her own problems that she was unable to be a nurturing, protecting mother to her children. How then were Rena and her sister to embark on developing their own womanhood? They hated their only female role model figure—yet the person they hated was still their mother, and along with their hate was a need for love. The sisters had strong ambivalent feelings about their mother, which became the attitude they later adopted toward their own sexuality: Rena became a compulsive overeater, her sister a nymphomaniac.

Rena, like most girls, reached a stage of adolescence when sexuality could no longer be denied. At this point, we must look at the importance of the menstrual cycle in relation to body-image and femininity. Premenstrual swelling of her breasts reminded Rena each month of her undeniable womanhood. The monthly bleeding also affirmed that she was a woman, a potential mother.

At the same time, Rena's adolescent sexual desires were growing with the normal strength of that stage of development. Her attitudes toward womanhood and genital sex were so confused and ambivalent that she did not dare seek sexual gratification appropriate to her genital development. Instead she returned to pregenital satisfactions on the oral level. For Rena and women like her oral gratification served as a mask for her genital desires.

Rena's mother provided her with an unhealthy model for womanhood and with the example of compulsive oral gratification through alcohol. Instead of being a compulsive drinker, Rena became a compulsive eater. We have had other patients whose parents had problems with alcoholism; since the primary model the parent offered for dealing with the world was oral the child grew up with that primitive example as the one to follow.

Rena was not arrested in either the oral or the anal stage of development. She had continued to grow and to develop, both physically and emotionally, to the genital stage. Her use of oral gratification was an aberration of her genital sexuality, and her overeating had all the energy and compelling force of a strong adolescent sex drive.

Since Rena's overeating was a mask for her genital sexuality, overeating elicited the same negative feelings in her that womanhood did: she hated food, and ate it angrily and quickly. She felt "dirty" when she ate, and in fact would let her hair, body, and clothes get dirty when she binged. She became as "bad" and "dirty" as she felt her mother to be. She chose junk food—the junkier the better. In that way, the food better fit her sense of its sinfulness.

Rena eventually married. A coldly disciplinarian older man, her husband expected intercourse as a duty, not as a true sexual outlet. This suited Rena's own denial of sexual gratification and her confused sexual drive. Mothering became an exaggerated part of her life: she had six children, closely spaced. Even with a house full of children, Rena mothered any stray animal that came along. She was preoccupied with thoughts of the children she had lost in miscarriages, with orphans in other countries, with puppies, kittens, and even plants and flowers that needed special tending.

Rena's overeating gave her the appearance of a pregnant woman. The junk foods she craved, high in carbohydrates, caused considerable fluid retention. When she felt fat and pregnant she was able to maintain a hazy concept of herself as a woman. But with it also was the feeling of being dirty and disgusting—like her mother. Thus, through her overeating she tried to express the love and hate she felt for her mother and for her own womanhood.

Whenever Rena tried to diet she felt she had stopped "sinning." She felt "clean" and took care of her personal appearance. At such times she would control her moods and keep her thoughts rational and cold, not letting any of her femininity drive her. Dieting for her was associated with the good, masculine, controlled part of herself. With dieting Rena knew she was not her mother.

It is important here to discuss Rena's feeling that overeating is bad and can be its own punishment: she eats until she hurts. Overeating for her has a masochistic quality, filled with self-hate and self-punishment. She hates the part of herself that is like her mother and punishes herself for being in some way like the woman she despises.

Rena was very afraid of her strong drives, which she felt but did not understand. It was easier for her to deal with her confusing and conflicting feelings if she divided her ambivalence: sometimes she was the gorger and sometimes she was the dieter. Overeating and dieting became cyclical. Whatever part of her cycle Rena was in, we always saw in her body the terribly exaggerated amount of blocked energy. The pent-up sexuality—never satisfied, always given substitute outlets through caring for children and animals—lived buried in the temperament of this huge woman. Rena had acquired hundreds of pounds of flesh to try to contain her buried feelings. None of the food satisfied her, however: under the mounds of fat she still felt a fire raging.

Anger is a problem for Rena. She knows there is something inside her clamoring to get out. Since she cannot identify it accurately, she suspects that *any* strong feeling may be the powerful thing she is so afraid of. She shared with us fantasies of how powerful her anger could be: she imagined herself tearing down a fireplace because she was angry with the people sitting in front of it. Weaker images were not in her fantasy. (She did not imagine crawling into the fireplace, for example.) It was instead a powerful, driven fantasy of destroying the whole structure. If the opening of the fireplace may be said to contain some female symbolism, then we know Rena needed to tear it apart.

It is appropriate to consider here what this bizarre case means in relation to obese persons in general. Rena's story raises questions about sexual attitudes that ought to be clarified. An overeater reading this book and attempting to explore his or her feelings about sexuality might ask the following:

"Does it bother me to be very much like a member of my own sex (i.e., very feminine or very masculine)?"
"Do I enjoy sexual intercourse or is it simply a duty?"

(Some patients in this cluster refrain from sexual intercourse completely.)
"Do I hate food but still overeat and stuff myself with a
vengeance?"
"Do I feel truly sinful when I overeat?"

Rena is an extreme example of a genital cluster overeater, yet much of her behavior is simply an exaggeration
of the behavior of other persons in this category.

BETH: THE INFERTILE OVEREATER

Beth is another patient whose eating problem reflects
characteristics of the genital cluster. Unlike Rena, however, her problem is not so extreme and therefore the
reader may be able to identify with her more easily.

Beth, now thirty-five, feels her eating problem did not
appear until she was twenty-five years old. At twenty-five
she married and waited to become pregnant. When she did
not conceive she began to question not only her fertility
but her femininity as well. She went to a fertility clinic for
a work-up, which she experienced as one of the most trying events of her life. When questioned directly about her
feelings concerning womanhood, Beth began to cry. She
recalled that her mother (with whom, she stated, she had
always had a good relationship) used to tell her that childbearing was the essence of womanhood.

It was during Beth's fertility work-up that she began to
overeat, gaining about thirty pounds over her previous
ideal weight. Over the past ten years she has kept that
extra weight, although dieting brings it down sporadi-
cally. Beth finds she is particularly depressed when she
thinks about her infertility and about more work-ups in
the future. When depressed, she feels herself to be especially fat, with the body-image of a woman much heavier
than she actually is.

It is intriguing to speculate on the fact that Beth's body-image is that of a pregnant woman who will not be able to deliver her offspring. Feeling fat is obviously connected to her juvenile conception of womanhood. Yet being fat is also a loss: she intuitively knows she has missed other parts of womanhood. As an adult, Beth has a more instinctively mature concept of what femininity may be. She senses that making herself thirty pounds overweight is part of a juvenile preoccupation with womanhood as childbearing. The loss of female sensuality and attractiveness is felt in her depression. There is a conflict between her inner, primitive image of carrying a baby and an adult concept of a fuller female experience. Beth feels ambivalent about being overweight. Her mixed feelings are similar to Rena's ambivalence about overeating. The positive aspect of overeating for Rena was that she sought sexual gratification in this way; the negative feeling was that overeating was dirty. For Beth the positive aspect was the feeling of being bloated and pregnant, while the negative aspect was in missing the sensuality of being female.

Beth's mother had instructed her to give up sexuality in place of maternity. The extra thirty pounds made her feel that she was listening to her mother's teachings. Dieting always made her feel naughty, slim, and sensuous. Those sexy feelings brought a new problem: Beth wondered if her husband would be "enough" for her. Whenever she dieted, she had fantasies about affairs with other men. In dieting she was not doing what her mother had taught her to do: she wasn't pregnant and she wasn't fat; she was thin and sexy and dangerous. There was more to being a woman than having babies—this Beth sensed whenever she lost some weight.

Their conflicting feelings toward obesity and food indicate that Beth and Rena both are struggling with ambivalence about sexual satisfaction. The positive feelings they experience are largely instinctual, part of the biological development of women. Their sexual drive suggests to them, on an unconscious level, that adult sexual relations would be pleasurable. The media, TV, books, magazines, popular song lyrics, also suggest this pleasure. But rooted in their past is the notion that sexual gratification on an adult level would be a negative, distasteful, naughty, or sinful experience. Both women, therefore, experience a great deal of anxiety about their adult sexuality.

Most genital cluster overeaters, like Beth and Rena, received some forms of satisfaction at early points in their development. As adults they yearn for these early forms of satisfaction that their mothers offered (or suggested existed) whenever they are faced with excessive frustrations. When their sexual relationships are frustrated on a genital level, they return to the oral level.

In Beth's case there is a clear correlation between the thirty pounds she gained (ironically, just about the weight women gain during a normal pregnancy) and the issue of her fertility. Of course, many women have fertility problems without such a weight gain. Being a woman includes having babies. But it hopefully also includes the ability to sustain an intimate sexual relationship, to give and receive genital pleasure. If these things were not part of her mother's life, then Beth could not readily learn about them. Beth expected the primary pleasure of womanhood would come with pregnancy. Disappointed at not achieving this, she began to overeat and in so doing returned to an earlier source of pleasure—oral gratification. Too ambivalent to be fulfilled by the healthier gratification of mature womanhood, she returned to the kinds of satisfactions that suffice for the immature, pregenital personality.

LEE: THE LITTLE MOM

The case of Lee illustrates some other characteristics frequently found in genital cluster overeaters. Lee also has many of the traits found in the anal cluster, emphasizing our contention that no individual has characteristics that fit into one cluster alone.

Lee, an intelligent, rather homely forty-year-old woman, presented herself to us with a desire to lose weight. Her weight history indicated that she did indeed have an eating problem and that she was significantly overweight from six to twelve years of age. Her weight was not a problem again until she was twenty, after which it continued to increase.

What happened to Lee when she was six years old? She recalls that around that time her life seemed to be highly involved in an interesting relationship with her younger sister. Lee's family adored the beautiful younger sibling, who had been born when Lee was three. Lee, neither attractive nor cuddly, was nevertheless clever and learned to win the admiration of her family by her ability to look after her baby sister. By the time Lee was six she had firmly established herself as a kind of "little mom" to her sister. This maternal quality became central to her identity.

As Freud and many others have made clear, the basic roots of sexuality and sexual identity develop early in childhood. At six, Lee already had the roots of her own unique concept of womanhood. During this period, like other girls her age, she was competing for her father's attention. This phenomenon (called the Oedipal conflict) has strong sexual connotations and puts the little girl in a threatening position—open conflict with her mother. Since the mother is a powerful and important figure to every child, the daughter does not truly wish to compete with her or to win the contest because she does not want to lose her mother. Nevertheless, there is still the desire in her to gain the attention of her father.

The Oedipal conflict is classically resolved by the little girl through her eventual identification with the mother, permitting her to possess the father vicariously. Identifying with her mother's femininity therefore becomes central to her own sexual identity. Through imitation of her mother's female ways, the child hopes to get the same attention and affection her mother gets from the father.

Lee had difficulty in resolving her Oedipal conflict because her father did not show her affection. He related more to his adorable, cuddly, younger daughter. Lee learned to win his appreciation indirectly—by helping the family care for her little sister. She became the giver: femininity became linked to the concept of nurturing.

At this early age Lee's understanding of how to give nurturance was closely related to food. This is not surprising, since her own experience with the feeding, nurturing mother was not too far behind her. She began to feed and care for her sister, and even prepared some of the meals. Between the ages of six and twelve, much of Lee's energy was tied up in mothering her sister. It was precisely during these years that Lee became overweight.

Lee was acting out the role of the selfless mother who gives to her children and asks nothing in return. When the children of such mothers are ready to reject their mothers' overinvolvement with them, they must reject the nurturance. Dieting is linked to rejection of mother, just as overeating is linked with the need for her. Diet is central today for all the grown children who eat compulsively when they crave the nurturance of their mothers.

When Lee was twelve, her sister had reached the more independent stage that begins at about nine. Lee was able to become more involved with her own peer group now. During this time she was largely free from being a mother to her younger sister. Her self-concept as a girl was able to attach itself to other new feelings; she lost weight and in fact maintained a normal weight throughout her adolescence.

Knowing this pattern of her early childhood, we can now try to understand why Lee's weight did not remain normal. She was courted by a young man who was bright, handsome, and demanding. This man, Peter, had always been a taker. Lee was basically a giver—so Lee gave and Peter, like her little sister, took. His psychological immaturity played right into hers: her underlying pathology, her need to be the all-giving mother, meshed with the weaknesses of his own personality.

After Lee and Peter were married, Lee became overweight again. In their sexual relations Lee was unable to achieve climax. Climax requires the ability to receive pleasure. Since Lee had always been a giver, she could not readily accept the pleasure of orgasm. Her underlying self-image prevented normal adult sexual gratification. By choosing Peter, she was re-enacting the pattern of her early family life: with him she could be a woman in the only way she knew how to be one—as a mother-figure.

Lee and Peter eventually had a baby. Inevitably, it became the main object of Lee's nurturing impulses; Peter could no longer be the prime taker. He was not able to tolerate this change and retaliated by rejecting Lee sexually. Lee's self-esteem was shattered. She lived under these demeaning conditions for years, however—caring for her family, spending a great deal of time preparing meals, enduring her husband's sexual rejection, and growing obese. When separation became inevitable for Lee and Peter, she sought professional help.

At this point Lee was able to accept the need to diet. She no longer had to keep trying to be a super-mom to her husband and her children. Being a woman no longer had to be so completely linked to giving nurturance. Along with dieting, Lee could now begin to learn to ask that her own needs be met. For the further development of her genital sexuality, it was necessary for her to learn to ask for—and receive—pleasure.

This was the beginning of real emotional growth for Lee. Until then she had never done anything for herself, only for others. She began therapy and realized that her "selfish" giving behavior had been a form of feeding herself. Hungry to receive, she had denied the need, yet had been giving herself food secretly, compulsively, and excessively. Getting therapy for herself meant getting emotional support. Her therapist was a woman who helped Lee to explore other avenues of femininity instead of nurturance of self-sacrifice on behalf of others.

Lee's strongly ingrained attitude toward food centered around its use as a symbol of caring. However, she also had natural biological desires to be gratified herself. Because her sexual relationship with her husband was not gratifying, she had to give to herself—which she did in the only way she knew how. Lee nurtured herself—albeit self-destructively—through eating.

Lee's sexuality had not developed during her genital stage. She sought gratification in nurturance and feeding, a more primitive form of sexual pleasure. She was not able to masturbate, but instead fed herself—her substitute expression for sexual self-gratification.

Lee had ambivalent feelings about the food she gave herself: she felt she was supposed to be the mother and the giver only. The food she took for herself she ate secretly and guiltily. But she desperately needed to replenish her supplies because she was being drained by meeting the needs of her children and husband. By eating more and more, she grew larger and larger, so that she might have more to give. Lee's full breasts were to her the symbol of her femininity: she was the well-supplied mother. Eating excessively was not only a selfish and greedy act, but a selfless act, for in so doing she was able to feed herself and keep the large bosom that signified that she could feed others.

When Lee lost Peter, she began to attend more closely to her own needs. She had no further need for such full breasts. After the shock of separation, she was able to diet. For her dieting was a way of giving up nurturing femininity. She began to deny herself the kind of distorted femininity she had grown up with. Rena and Beth also used a controlled diet to deny forms of femininity that had become disturbing to them. In all these cases dieting means finally denying the unhealthy forms of gratification that had been sought earlier.

Most of Lee's problems with overeating place her firmly in the genital cluster. "Does this person feel sinful when overeating?" Lee kept her sin a secret, hiding the fact that the family giver was gorging herself. "Is sexual intercourse a source of pleasure or a duty for this person?" Lee did not enjoy intercourse; it was something she gave to Peter without any thought of enjoyment for herself. "Does this woman feel uncomfortable with the idea of being very feminine?" Indeed, Lee had strong, ambivalent feelings about her femininity.

Some of Lee's problems with overeating stem from problems of the anal cluster. In part, at least, her overeating was a symptom of low self-esteem. When her first husband rejected her, her weight increased. This was not because she was sexually frustrated, but because she felt herself to be a failure. Binging with food helped her to dull these feelings. At the same time the pain her body endured through overeating was a way of punishing herself for losing her husband.

DAVE: BEING A MAN

In our respective practices we have found that in general more women than men suffer from obesity. (We will try to understand this phenomenon better when later considering social factors in the development of obesity.) And although fewer men fit into the genital cluster, it is important to study their case histories as well. Characteristically, these men became overweight during adolescence, turning—like the women we have discussed—to food instead of sex for instinctual gratification. Dave was such a young man.

As a sixteen-year-old high school student Dave weighed

250 pounds. His mother was a successful business woman who ran her own store. His father was a soft-spoken, gentle man who helped his wife run her business. He accommodated her needs so their store and home could be run more easily. One way of doing this was by taking the family out to dinner after the store closed. In this way, Dave's father represented the nurturing, food-providing partner.

When Dave reached his teens, he was making great achievements as a student. His school record was quite brilliant as he spent more and more time at his desk. But he gained weight and had no muscle tone.

Dave's father was a passive and non-athletic man; the drive and aggression in the family all came from his mother's side. She weighed a formidable 186 pounds, about 75 pounds more than her short frame should have carried. Thus strength for Dave was perceived in the female parent, not the male. In acquiring strength for himself he made himself a receptacle—of information and of food. His hours of studying also became hours of snacking, as he took in calories along with facts. He did not at any time during his adolescence act out any of his impulses to become aggressive or sexually involved. These impulses were kept buried under the layers of fat his body was accumulating.

Dave came into treatment to lose weight during a summer vacation. On a very strict diet he was able to lose weight rapidly, as young men frequently can. During the first two weeks, in fact, he lost almost twenty-five pounds. His treatment program also included exercises for physical conditioning and for eliciting emotions.

As his body changed rapidly and strange new feelings began to express themselves, Dave stopped dieting. He felt confusion as to who and what he was. He began to think of himself and his masculinity as some sort of evil or monstrous force. His parents were encouraged to get psychological help for their son.

This was not a success story. Dave's parents insisted that

his overweight was due to his habit of snacking while studying and not to any more serious problems. Dave regained his weight and left treatment. He did not get professional help to find a way of being aggressive and male, but continued instead to channel his creative mind into his scholastic work and intellectual accomplishments.

MORRIS: THE LITTLE PHALLUS

We will now present a more extreme case of a man who belongs to the genital cluster. The bizarre story of Morris clearly depicts the link between obesity and distorted sexuality. Body-image and sexual identity are usually far subtler issues than they appear here.

Morris, thirty-five and about 5'7" tall, presented himself to us weighing 350 pounds. His masculinity was so deeply troubled that he surrounded himself with such male sex symbols as dirty jokes, pornographic objects, foul language, as well as more socially acceptable objects such as cigars, pipes, oversized pens and pencils, and ornate walking canes.

When taking a dietary history we found that Morris did eat compulsively but in a very idiosyncratic way: he reported episodes of stuffing himself with foods shaped like penises. He frequently ate a dozen cannoli at a time or an equal quantity of frankfurters, still frozen.

When questioned about his sex life, Morris admitted that in his youth he had been terribly ashamed of his penis, feeling it to be much smaller than most. He entered the army but found himself miserable because he was constantly worrying about hiding his penis for fear of being ridiculed by the other men. In fact, Morris's penis was small. Because of his obesity, however, the penis had become almost lost in rolls of fat. He had eventually married, but had never had intercourse with his wife.

Morris agreed to enter treatment with the aid of psycho-

logical counseling as well as diet. Some of the psychodynamics of his case were soon revealed. His father had
seemed to him powerless and controlled by Morris's
strong-minded mother. He eventually became ill and was
confined to a wheelchair—thus strengthening Morris's
view of his father as totally dependent on his mother. Morris saw his mother as a very hostile and demanding
woman. He felt she had little understanding of others, was
very narcissistic, and very controlling. As a grown man,
Morris says he seldom actually sees her or talks to her any
longer, but thoughts of his mother are almost always with
him.

Morris was never good at making a living, although he
lived fairly well on large sums of money borrowed from a
brother who ran a successful business. When Morris entered treatment his wife was working while he collected
unemployment insurance. He spent his days in the house,
and when his wife came home from work he sent her out
to get him food.

The strangeness of this marriage can best be understood
if one sees it as a repetition of the dynamics Morris saw
between his own mother and father. Morris has obviously
identified with his mother—demanding, controlling, and
narcissistic. His wife reacts to him in the weak, compliant
way that his own father had behaved toward Morris's
mother.

Morris is obviously very ambivalent about the role he
takes and has found many ways to overcompensate for his
underlying lack of male identification. He maintains a
pose of brash masculinity that by its very exaggerated
nature betrays its superficiality. He swears incessantly, for
example, and talks about seducing women, though he has
never done so. He gladly offers vivid descriptions of how
"horny" he is all the time. His pockets are full of phallic
symbols—king-size cigars, large pipes, and pens.

This behavior is mainly bravado; Morris's male identity
is a big, flashy show. His real sexual identity is kept under

control when he acts the part of a macho male. It is when he is binging that his true self begins to be revealed and that his deeper desires come to the surface: he loses his pseudo-interest in women, along with his symbolic pride in his personal appearance. Like his mother, he stays at home and becomes more demanding and bossy when he goes on one of his binges.

When Morris's body swells up he claims he looks pregnant. He feels his appetite is ravenous—that is why he cannot wait for the frozen frankfurters to defrost before devouring them. His binging has the intensity and urgency of sexual passion. These are stories he also likes to tell: it feels sexy to him to tell other men about his binges.

As we study this case, we see the striking similarity between Morris and Rena. Rena is Morris's female counterpart, so to speak. She is an extreme example of the female genital overeater who felt "dirty" during her junk-food binges. She too became unkempt and ravenous when binging. Their sexuality, which seemed perverse to them, found expression in an orgy of eating.

We must look here at the receptive characteristics of femininity. Because of both biological and cultural differences between men and women, passivity and receptivity are usually considered feminine qualities. The female sexual organs are internal and so constructed as to receive the male organ. It is not surprising, therefore, that binging with strong sexual overtones takes on a feminine quality, since the entire body becomes a receptive organ during the act of eating.

Eating is also intimately connected with breast and bottle feeding. Overeating can simulate a bloated feeling in the body, similar to premenstrual fluid retention or to the condition of pregnancy. It follows that overeating for a man like Morris can easily be transformed into an expression of his female sexual identity.

As with Dave, who also had problems with his sexual identity, any weight reduction program for extreme cases like Morris's must afford an opportunity to come to terms with the question of sexual identity. The confusion within such men as to whether their sexuality is male or female is responsible for much of their eating behavior.

Morris's case affords us the clearest picture of a confused sexual identity: whether he dieted or binged, he was still the same confused person. When he dieted he controlled his most passionate behavior but concentrated much of his energy on collecting jewelry and flashy clothes instead. His confusion was especially evident when he once impulsively traded his costly pipe collection for a gaudy silver and turquoise bracelet, exchanging typically masculine symbols for feminine ones.

During his months of dieting while in treatment with us Morris's collection of jewelry grew; indeed, much of his money was spent on rings, bracelets, buckles, etc. At the doctor's office he ritualistically took off each piece of the heavy jewelry before stepping onto the scale, frequently remarking that he felt like a flashy female prostitute. His sexual identity was as confused as ever, even during dieting, although he had more control of his female sexuality during these non-binging periods. He was able to keep control of his inner self with an external show of dress and with compulsive collecting of expensive objects.

SUMMARY

In this chapter we have presented five cases illustrating the psychological problems of the genital cluster overeater—problems revolving around distorted expressions of sexual desire and around sexual identity. Diet for such persons is only an artificial means of controlling their needs. The diet may be necessary, and in fact often provides a respite from the acting out of inner turmoil. But it is usually short-lived and sometimes even part of a binge-diet cycle.

Those who belong to this category have a special task before they can diet successfully: they must attempt to explore and understand their feelings about sexuality. This is not an easy job, and generally requires professional help and guidance. When diet is the only tool used by the genital cluster overeater, it is at best a very temporary treatment of a deep-seated symptom. If a diet is part of the binge cycle, it probably represents repentance after a "sinful" eating orgy. The doctor who simply prescribes a diet for such a patient becomes an accomplice and helps to maintain this compulsive cycle. When overeating is symptomatic of underlying problems in the genital character development, the responsible doctor must first attend to this issue. As it is resolved, dieting will **follow** more easily and more successfully.

6

The Adolescent-Onset Overeater

THE DYNAMICS

Some overeaters develop their eating problems during adolescence. During these years young men and women are trying to "find themselves." The identity conflicts they encounter usually have their roots in earlier developmental stages. Overeaters who belong to this cluster are frequently reminiscent of overeaters who had oral, anal, or genital conflicts, but if their eating problems arise during puberty there are characteristics which separate them from members of the other clusters. By understanding these particular characteristics, we will see that adolescent-onset overeaters must be treated differently from the others.

Adolescents are searching for a connection between their early childhood sense of self and the possibilities of that same self existing in the adult world. They carry with them the degree of trust that they developed, as infants, in the world and in themselves. In addition, they carry into adolescence feelings they have developed about their own initiative or lack of it, and feelings about their own and the opposite sex.[1] They are primarily preoccupied with defining themselves, whereas during the preceding genital stage they usually defined themselves by identifying with father or mother. For a teenager this identification is no longer adequate; he wants to become his own person. In order to find himself, so to speak, he must reject the very person he identified with in the first place.

An important characteristic of adolescence, then, is rebellion. The normal teenager now seeks his own group, a society of peers, to bolster his rebellion against the values of his parents. Finding his new identity involves a struggle against the parental identity. The way he handles that struggle may range from surrender—"the blob"—to violent self-assertion—"the rebel." His ability to compromise depends upon character developments that preceded his adolescence: the teenager with severe problems is usually either over-rebellious or over-submissive.[2]

Teenagers are narcissistically preoccupied with their own image. The search for identity inevitably requires such self-absorption. Other people are seen as images, too: an adolescent does not deal with people as people, but rather treats them like stock characters. This person is a "nurd," that one is a "turkey." Teenage slang is fraught with such language because of the great image-consciousness and narcissistic preoccupation of the stage. Searching for their own self-image, adolescents label and categorize everyone around them; those who win their approval are "in" people, those who do not are "out."

Narcissistic, viewing the world largely in terms of how it relates to him, the teenager struggles to consolidate his self-image. If the struggle is an ongoing one that is still unresolved by the stage of adulthood, it is likely to show up in eating problems as well as in other areas. Even if a patient comes to the doctor with a weight problem at the age of fifty, the unresolved adolescent problems are still identifiable if the overeater is narcissistically preoccupied with himself and his image, if he is still having trouble with social roles and social restrictions, if he is over-rebellious and outspoken or over-submissive and quiet. This person still is not sure what he wants out of life. He may have jumped from job to job or mate to mate, and sexual problems are likely. Significantly, his self-image and body-image tend to be inconsistent with reality.

Swinging from rebellion to submission and back again, being narcissistic and concerned with images—this is the normal course of events during the adolescent years when young people are attempting to deal with two new subjects: sex and society. It is the appropriate time in their lives to be figuring out sex roles because sexual maturity takes place in these years; it is also time to understand social roles because they are leaving childhood and entering adulthood.

The adolescent must cope with his new-found sexuality and incorporate it into his self-image. Some degree of confusion about body-image is common at this time when genital development and hormonal changes create bursts of energy and strong impulses along with bodily growth. For young people who have gone through the oral, anal, and genital stages with adequate success, it is less difficult to deal with this surge of sexuality in adolescence. But for those who carry with them poorly resolved problems from those earlier stages, the new impulses are hard to accept. The adolescent troubled in this way is frightened of the changes occurring in both his personality and his body. Frightened by what his own body seems to be desiring, he develops barriers against these new impulses and refuses to accept his body's signals. Instead, he clings to a body-image that feels safer, even if it is inconsistent with his body's desires or its actual physical condition. He (often she) may avoid sex or go to the opposite extreme of sexual promiscuity. Either way, his aberrant behavior creates a barrier against genuine knowledge or acceptance of his impulses. His self-image is distorted, and this basic adolescent period of development goes unresolved.[3]

BOBBIE: THE 37-YEAR-OLD TEENAGE JUNK FOOD ADDICT

Let us now look at the case of an adolescent-onset over-eater from our own files. Bobbie was a woman who came to us at the age of thirty-seven. She was about thirty pounds overweight, but since her body-image was some-what distorted she felt herself to be about fifty pounds overweight. She talked a great deal about herself and her feelings, finding tremendous pleasure in such conversa-tion, to a degree suggesting a narcissistic preoccupation. She seemed almost like a teenager—full of strong, rebel-lious attitudes. She was quite sincere and intense, and could talk about what she felt in very explicit terms.

Bobbie told us that her mother was an authoritarian, cold, and compulsive woman who ran the house and thor-oughly controlled the domestic scene. Good, wholesome food was of paramount importance and all junk food was forbidden. In Bobbie's words, "she taught me the seven essential foods before the alphabet." By contrast, her fa-ther was unassertive and warm. Bobbie described him as an "ineffectual Spencer Tracy."

When Bobbie became a teenager, she rebelled violently against her mother, trying to define herself in terms of opposites. Her mother was morally puritanical; Bobbie became flirtatious, began sexual intercourse at fourteen, and brought her black boyfriend home to shock her mother. Her mother wanted her to be a nurse or a teacher; she became an artist. At the age of thirty-one she had a falling out with her mother and has refused to speak to her ever since. The rebellion is still going on at age thirty-seven.

Bobbie is a woman with unresolved adolescent problems

that she re-enacts continually. Even though she was twenty-eight when she married, she perpetuated her rebellious drama by choosing a man who was strong, cold, and compulsive—just like her mother. The marriage lasted three years and ended in her demand for a separation.

Eating problems began for Bobbie in her teens when she started to use junk food as part of her rebellion. Junk food gives her a feeling of her own strength: when she is under stress or is called upon to do something difficult or requiring independent action, Bobbie binges on junk food. Her overeating at these times is compulsive behavior that she cannot control.

If we look at Bobbie's early history, we can understand something of her eating problem. Her mother was cold and could not give Bobbie warmth with her nurturance. Since the mother is the first giver of food, there is a lifelong link from infancy on between food and mother. Bobbie's mother carefully controlled all the food her daughter was allowed to eat, always stressing wholesomeness. The connection between food and mother was very clearly delineated for the child.

When Bobbie rebelled from her mother, she naturally rejected her mother's food. She began to eat a lot of junk food, which became symbolic of her own choice, her own identity. She had to separate from her overbearing mother, and she used food as one of her ways of doing this. At critical times, when she needed to feel that she was strong, that she could act on her own, she sought strength and self-identity through junk food. Her identity became clearer to her if she could "fill up" on her own choice of food.

It is important to realize that as a teenager Bobbie was not in touch with any true sense of self, nor did she have a high self-esteem. We postulate that her adolescent problem was related to an earlier stage of development that must have been problematical for her—the anal stage, when she ought to have been able to develop a feeling of initiative and self-esteem.

This case provides clear evidence of the link between early developmental problems at the anal stage and their adolescent recurrence. Bobbie's mother was rigid and Bobbie's toilet training was presumably rigid. Her meals were on a fixed schedule and she ate only "good" foods, not being permitted the freedom to explore her own appetities or impulses. By the time Bobbie became a teenager, she had not developed an inner trust in her own strength or worth. To feel separate and/or strong as an individual she had to overeat and overrebel. Instead of finding compromise solutions, she was driven to extremes.

Bobbie needed props, such as junk food, in order to feel strong because her basic self-esteem and initiative were so weak. She flaunted her independence as if to say "See, I do what I want to do. I have initiative." She overdid it because she had to deny to herself that in fact she did not have initiative. Her teenage rebellion was a violent, angry denial of her childhood dependency on an extremely controlling mother.

Bobbie's problems have not been resolved. She married a man who was like her mother, gave into him for a while, then rebelled—first on the subject of budgeting their expenses. To this day she cannot—will not—account for her own expenses. Now a divorced woman, Bobbie continues her compulsive overeating of junk food, still needing that rebellious defense to protect her tenuous identity.

How should we treat Bobbie's eating problem? If we prescribe a diet for her and tell her which foods are "good" and which are "bad," we will surely become aligned with her mother. This would cause tremendous anxiety for Bobbie.[4] She needs support in finding what her own true appetites, hungers, and impulses really call for. Like many teenagers, she can probably accept such support best from a peer group rather than an authority figure. Such support would help to bolster her self-esteem, because she would find strength in people whose images she can identify as being closer to her own. Thus, group therapy and group dieting may be the most helpful means of treating an overeater like Bobbie.

Fusion and Rebellion

The issues of the adolescent-onset cluster are all central to the development of a person's separate adult identity. Some, like Bobbie, get stuck in the rebellious stages of this development. Others submit, abandon their separate adult identity, and remain childishly fused with a parent's identity. In either the over-rebellious or the over-submissive solution, genuine personal feelings of strength are missing.

Very often a young person comes to the end of his or her adolescence without having fully developed a strong self-identity. When it is time to leave the parental home and enter new sexual or social roles, the going may be rough and there are often some difficult transitional months or years ahead. It is not unusual for weight gain or overeating to develop during such stressful times.

Our medical files show, for example, many cases of young women from tight-knit, warm homes who move away for the first time when they marry, and who in their first year of married life gain thirty pounds. We also see many college students who, leaving home for the first time, gain five pounds the first six weeks they are away at school. This underscores the strong connection many people make between the act of feeding and mother. The weight gain may be temporary, while the young persons learn new coping mechanisms for their adult lives. But if there existed a basic problem of early fusion of identity between parent and child, then the need and the yearning for nurturance is not readily resolved, and overeating often becomes a long-term problem.

One common solution to identity problems is marriage. For young girls especially, marriage represents an opportunity to fuse with a new person when it is time to leave the original parental home. Such young girls hope that their new husbands will help define them, tell them who and what they are. Since husbands are never likely to be the same as indulgent parents, their hunger for fusion is not satisfied. Nevertheless, the primitive connection between parental care and food is always there. Overeating is an attempt to satisfy the unfilled need for fusion with the longed-for nurturing and supporting conditions of earlier days. Unfortunately, however, while food may symbolize fusion, it never really *is* fusion, and so compulsive overeating never truly satisfies the hunger for identity.

Treatment of adults who are still struggling with these adolescent problems can be very stormy. For example, the woman who has submitted her identity to a controlling husband must rebel within that relationship in order to define herself on her own terms. If she did in fact choose her husband in order to fuse as a way of defining her identity, she must see that relationship for what it is: a reenactment of her childhood submission to parental authority.

When questions of submission and fusion are prominent in the case of the adolescent-onset overeater, the roots of the problem are to be found in the oral stage of development. In spite of those early problems, growth continued until adolescence, when overeating became a prop and no true solutions to teenage problems evolved. The post-adolescent is then left with a sense of inadequate understanding of self. Even as an adult, he or she is still searching for a self, still trying to be "somebody."

To be arrested at the oral stage of development is to be like Dolly, the woman described in Chapter 3. Because of Dolly's total fusion with her mother, she could not develop any trust in herself and could take no genuine independent action. She was not aware of her own needs, nor did she ever develop even a childhood identity of her own.

In contrast to Dolly, the adolescent-onset overeater who has had some difficulty in oral development went on to function well in the world as a pre-teen, developing some sense of self—although this feeling is not sufficient to withstand the real separation from parents that should come during adolescence. If submission to parents becomes the chosen solution, it is accompanied by uneasy feelings of stagnation and avoidance of growth and by some brief rebellious questioning, none of which ever bothered Dolly. The adolescent-onset overeater is plagued by thoughts about his or her own identity, which contributes to the narcissistic quality of their behavior.

In the case of an adolescent-onset overeater, there is a correlation between how the teenager deals with food and how he deals with other aspects of that stage of growth. Bobbie rejected her mother's good food and gorged herself with junk food; her eating behavior was as over-rebellious as the rest of her behavior at that period. Submissive teenagers gorge themselves with food when they yearn for fusion and resist the growing separation with parents; their eating behavior and their longing for "home" represent the denial of an emerging independent self.

The phenomenon of anorexia nervosa (most common in teenage girls) interests us here because it is one form of eating behavior which does *not* result in overeating or obesity. Instead, it represents a bizarre and extreme form of rejection: these girls reject food so totally that they often risk death by starvation. They reject the identification with their mothers when their pubescent bodies begin to develop wider hips, thighs, and breasts. They consider this fat and must reject it, and with it their femininity. With severe weight loss, their new hormonal balance is destroyed and menstruation—another despised symbol of femininity—stops.

Hilda Bruch has suggested that anorexics do not consider their identity their own.[5,6] She attributes this to, among other things, "the mother's superimposing on the child her own concept of the child's needs." The rejection of food is an extreme attempt to establish a separate identity from an all-powerful mother. The extreme nature of the rebellion bears witness to the extreme controllingness of the mother. Unfortunately, the rejection of food is an overly concrete gesture: at this stage it is the suffocating demands for conformity that should be rejected. Anorexics do not truly confront and challenge their mothers' values and beliefs. Instead, their rebellion is misdirected toward an almost total rejection of food that is sometimes fatal.

SUMMARY

Bobbie rejected her mother's "good" food and ate junk food. In the body of this thirty-seven-year-old woman was a teenager with problems. Rebellion against parents, narcissism, and distorted body image are classical adolescent problems. In dealing with the weight problem of an adolescent-onset overeater, one must deal with identity problems. Support and role models are best supplied by peer groups, as they usually are for adolescents. Group therapy and group dieting are frequently helpful in the treatment of this overeater.

7

The Adult-Onset Overeater

THE DYNAMICS

At times of stress, it is part of human nature to go back to behavior that once helped us to cope and that made us feel good. A classic example was observed when anthropologists entered a village in Africa where the inhabitants were still living a very isolated jungle existence. Children who had recently been weaned toddled back to their mothers when the strangers appeared and began to nurse at the exposed breasts. Their instinct was to return to the stage of development that had previously offered comfort and a successful way of dealing with stress.

When overeating begins during adulthood, it is often precipitated by some significant interruption or change in lifestyle or circumstance. Overeating becomes the pattern of behavior which the individual chooses as a way of dealing with stress—adjusting to his new needs or to the changes in the demands made by his environment.

Some adults merely overeat out of habit rather than

compulsively, and gain weight when their activity decreases with age and with a more sendentary lifestyle. Their treatment is simpler and usually more successful than that tailored for compulsive eaters, consisting of behavior modification techniques.

Not all adults search for adaptive forms of behavior. Overeating, for example, is common in our society. Some people eat to comfort themselves, and overeat without perceiving or taking into account the discomfort that ensues. Continual or compulsive overeating, in the face of unsolved problems, is maladaptive behavior: it may well be a reaction to disturbance or emotional tension, but it does not and can never adequately quell the disturbance or erase the tension. Many overweight adults deal with their problems by returning to the archaic solutions of infancy, childhood, or adolescence. Occasionally they find some comfort from this behavior, but most often the regression proves to be maladaptive, and their problems continue.

MILLIE: FRUSTRATION IN MARRIAGE

Millie came to us weighing 185 pounds at a height of 5'3". As usual, we asked her when she started gaining this weight. She said that weight had never been a real problem until after she underwent surgery for cancer of the cervix, five years earlier. The cancer was located in such a way that the surgeon found it necessary to remove only a portion of the cervix. Millie had been pronounced cured thereafter.

We also asked Millie if anything else had occurred in her life about five years ago. She told us that sexual relations with her husband had changed dramatically at that time because he feared that she might have a recurrence of the tumor (he had heard the statistic that women who have intercourse have a higher incidence of cervical cancer than women who do not). His fears for his wife's health, his tendency to be a worrier, and this piece of scientific information led him to the conclusion that he ought not to have sexual intercourse with his wife after her surgery.

Millie first mentioned her lack of intercourse over the past five years in an almost nonchalant tone. After further questioning on the subject, however, it became more obvious that she was indeed upset about this change in her life. She believed her husband was abstaining from sexual relations with her for her own good. Because she needed to trust him, she had not dared to ask a gynecologist for an opinion or advice on the subject. Yet Millie deeply missed the previous closeness she had shared with her husband.

Millie began to use overeating to fill up her sense of emptiness and loss. Though it was physical closeness and the feeling of oneness with her husband that she felt she had lost, it was food that she chose to replace her loss, returning to the infantile part of herself—the child trying to regain a feeling of unity with the world. Millie repeatedly attempted to orally incorporate the full feeling of being loved and satisfied. Yet although she ate and ate she never felt that satisfaction: her overeating was maladaptive, for it created no sense of fusion with her husband.

Many other women, when faced with sexual desertion or loss of a loved one, act in the way Millie did. Some become angry, but Millie suppressed all feelings of anger and doubt. She failed to take the initiative and seek medical advice on whether or not her husband's idea of linking intercourse with the spread of cancer was a correct one. Millie was a woman who feared her own anger and also avoided taking risks. During stressful periods she overate in a primitive attempt to fuse with her husband and as a way of suppressing her inner tensions and anger. Thus her overeating had both oral and anal qualities to it. Under stress she regressed to earlier stages of development, to behavior that once gave her comfort or escape. The disruption in her sexual relationship with her husband was a serious frustration to her, but because the anal part of her personality consistently required that she bury frustration and anger within herself, she had to push such feelings down with food.

We suggested that Millie bring her husband to the doctor's office on her next visit. At that time it was emphasized to the couple that medical science has not shown any relationship between intercourse and the spread of cervical cancer. Millie's husband seemed greatly relieved and expressed delight that he no longer had to refrain from intercourse with his wife. It appeared that he had had no other reason for his abstinence. Millie went home without a prescribed diet, having been told that with a rebirth of her sex life her weight might automatically return to normal.

Happily, Millie's sex life did have a rebirth and she gradually returned to her normal weight. As she said, "It just happened without really trying." Her personality did not change. In fact, she continued to have difficulty expressing her feelings and her anger. As she had done all of her life, she retained her tendency to overeat during times of stress. But whenever a particular set of problems was resolved, she was able to lose the extra pounds she had gained.

KENNETH: THE EX-FOOTBALL PLAYER

Kenneth's story will help clarify how to recognize an adult-onset overeater. He had been an outstanding football player in college. When he graduated he hoped for an offer to play professionally, but when this did not happen he entered his father's insurance business. Kenneth married the girl he had dated throughout college, and as he settled into his job and his marriage his physical activity decreased markedly. Nevertheless, he continued to eat as heartily as he had during his football days, steadily gaining weight over the next few years. Ken lost much of his former muscle bulk and his weight turned into "flab." As his life became more sedentary, his eating habits did not alter sufficiently to prevent a weight gain. Since Ken could not readily return to his previous level of energy expenditure, he would have to change his eating pattern if he wanted to lose weight.

What can be done for Kenneth and other adult-onset overeaters like him? In determining the proper treatment it is important to find out whether or not his eating is serving a significant function in his life, other than keeping him healthy and well nourished. In other words, is there an emotional reason for his eating behavior? Is he eating in order to suppress anger, to deal with a sexual problem, to cope with fears of separation or independence? Is an adult problem central to his overeating or does he belong to one of the earlier clusters?

Someone who appears to be an adult-onset overeater may in fact be using food to work out very early childhood problems. Even if he has not used overeating to handle these problems previously, it is important to know if the central issue behind the overeating is really an issue in his adult life or one that has been left unresolved from either infancy, childhood, or the teenage years. To determine whether an overeater belongs to the adult-onset cluster, it is necessary to ask a few pointed questions.

"Do you have trouble getting angry?" is a question aimed at opening up the discussion of emotional control. If this appears to be a difficult thing for the overeater to do, if anger and any strong emotions are confusing or upsetting to him, if he seems to avoid feelings or to get lost in them, a diagnosis in the anal cluster must be considered.

"Are you able to trust people?" "Do you enjoy trips, risks, gambling, adventures?" An oral cluster overeater is not able to trust himself, others, or the hands of fate. Consequently, he avoids these and other unpredictable or independent forms of behavior.

"Are you able to enjoy sex?" This question is not really

aimed at discovering the quantity of sexual experience or activity going on. Instead, it is designed to find out more about whether a patient's sexual fantasies are bizarre or suppressed, whether sex seems compulsive or prohibited, pleasurable or unsatisfying. If adolescent emotional development was traumatic or inhibited, the patient may be an adolescent-onset overeater who has never really found himself sexually or socially. There are people who are completely preoccupied with solving their "weight problem" as a way of postponing adulthood: like adolescents, they prefer to avoid the reality problems of adults and concern themselves instead with perpetually preparing to grow up. Such persons are likely to say that after they have lost weight they will be able to start a new career or job, or find somebody to love or marry. At the same time, they keep overeating, and so continue to postpone both the solution to their weight problem and the difficult confrontation with adult sexuality and social roles.

To determine more about Kenneth's reasons for overeating, we asked about his infancy and childhood. Kenneth reported that he had strict parents who constantly insisted he do what they wanted him to do. At around two, the anal stage of development, Ken ought to have evolved a sense of pride or self-esteem. The two-year-old would have been ready to develop an ability to feel and express his own emotions, including anger and self-assertion. In the food area these would have revolved around preferences for or disgust at certain foods. Kenneth evidently felt he had been forced by his parents into a particular mold to suit their own wishes and emotions. In the process of submitting to their will he became alienated from his own emotions, unsure of what he was actually feeling and of what he was supposed to be feeling. His anger at them became buried deep inside of him, unasserted and unexpressed.

As Kenneth grew, he found partial solutions to his emotional problems. He joined groups, for example, that were acceptable to his parents but which gave him some rules, regulations, and activities separate from theirs. He joined athletic teams in which the action tended to be aggressive, satisfying somewhat his desire to express his pent-up anger and aggression. As he tackled an opponent on the football field, he felt exhilaration. His buried anger, denied on the surface, could be structured and controlled according to the rules of the game. Nothing "bad" could happen to the angry two-year-old inside of him, because Ken the athlete was channeling his assertiveness and independence in behavior that accorded with the game's regulations; he felt safe.

When Kenneth graduated from college and did not get an offer to make a career out of professional sports, he lost the controlling structure that he had relied on by being the member of a team. He took the safest steps he could, entering his father's business and marrying his old college girlfriend. Defiant, self-assertive behavior had no sanctioned channel anymore, and Ken had to find a new way to keep his emotions under control now that he could no longer act them out on the football field. He felt panic when he was called upon to act independently, without rules to contain his energies. Life was not a game anymore: when he felt stress, frustration, or tension, he would have to keep them in.

He still ate the big meals he used to have as an athlete, but they were now not so much means of providing him with physical energy as desperate attempts to hold down his tension and quiet his frustration and anger. He submitted to the security of his father's business and the girl he had married by "swallowing" what they gave him. Kenneth began to eat compulsively, especially under stress. Before his graduation from college this had not been his pattern, since his athletic activities had allowed him to compensate for his emotional weaknesses. As an adult, therefore, his overeating was serving an emotional function in his life—a function that had not been necessary when he was younger and acting out his feelings through competitive sports.

In order to treat Kenneth, we had first to consider the problems arising from his anal personality. Though he seemed to have an adult-onset weight problem, Kenneth's problem is deeply rooted in the anal cluster. The difficulties he had had during the anal stage of his childhood development had produced the personality traits involved in his overeating as an adult.

Adult-onset overeaters can, like Ken, still have some uncomfortable feelings about basic trust, anger, independence, or even sexuality. But they have not been crippled during earlier developmental stages as he was. For them the central issues are latter-day changes in circumstances or a succession of crises that adult life has presented them with. Because the genuine adult-onset overeater has a far stronger personality than Ken's, he or she stands a greater chance of overcoming current eating problems.

WOMEN IN THE HOME

Adults, especially women, sometimes report the beginning of a weight problem after marriage.[1] When marriage is entered into as an attempt to solve an identity problem, it is not really an adult choice, for inside the adult is a hungry, needy infant or young person. Immature women are really longing for nurturing and supporting conditions for themselves that they failed to get in their original families. Marriage, however, will never satisfy all the unfilled needs and emotional hungers left over from childhood and adolescence.

The new husband is not in fact a new mother or father to be leaned on. The reverse is likely to be true: the new bride finds herself with someone to care for, cook for, clean for; *she* is responsible for providing nurturing and

124 • THE OVEREATERS

support. Her own left-over hungers may feel neglected, her appetite or need for supplies may be too voracious to be satisfied by what her husband offers. Many times she fills the emptiness inside her with the food she is cooking, or with the cold left-overs she has put in her refrigerator.

The fact that the young husband is out in the "world" building his new career often makes the marital situation more difficult. He is grappling with the difficult yet challenging task of solidifying his identity, and his climb has begun: the satisfactions, great and small, provided by his work achievements bolster his adult needs. His wife cannot always enjoy his triumphs, still hungry with unmet childhood needs.

Such women present more complicated problems than simple adult-onset overeaters, for clearly their weight gain is a symptom of emotional immaturity and not merely due to the fact that their marital status has changed. Because of this immaturity, their choice of a mate may have been inappropriate, and the marriage may be very unstable. If the woman attempts to solve her eating problem by getting professional help and "growing up," she may find that she wants to get out of the partnership her adolescent self got her into. Usually the emergence of the adult woman, through therapy or some other therapeutic experience, results in a stronger individual identity that can assert its needs in the home or in the world without filling up on food.

Motherhood is another point at which weight problems often begin.[2] When women begin this new part of their life cycle there is sometimes difficulty adjusting. The fact that they are literally involved in round-the-clock food preparations for their own hungry and needy infants makes it all the easier for them to nibble at food constantly. Frequently their difficulties are temporary, and when weight gain is a symptom of these stressful times, it can also be temporary—a problem that finds other solutions as the children grow older. New mothers often have much in common with new brides who try to feed their own emotional needs by overeating. In both cases, the young women are regressing to self-indulgent behavior: they are feeding the hungry girls inside themselves.

These new mothers are often struggling to cross the bridge between adolescence and adulthood. The hallmark of the latter is productivity or creativity in the adult roles of society. For many women, this can be a career or professional role, while for others it is having children. The adult's concern is for establishing and guiding the next generation—Erikson calls this generativity.[3] Emotionally immature mothers often overeat because they are not quite ready to become involved in the nurturing and support of others.

The weight problems of new brides and mothers are adult-onset because these specific conditions of adult life have triggered childhood or adolescent hungers. Women who have chosen the option of productivity or creativity in the home are most often affected not because they are less mature than women who work or pursue a career, but because so many of the symbols of love and care in their environment are food-oriented.

MELISSA: FAILURES AND REGRESSIONS

When Melissa came to us for her weight problem, she was thirty-four years old and weighed just over 250 pounds. The information she gave was that at twenty she had weighed 150 pounds; she stated too that at that time she felt she had not had an eating problem. When she was twenty-one she got married, and had her first child the next year.

When the baby was three months old, Melissa's husband was caught in an armed robbery. He attempted to escape and was killed in an auto accident while being chased by the police. Melissa seems never to have recovered from the

trauma and shame of her husband's death. She has difficulty expressing her anger at the circumstance of the accident. In fact, she seems to have difficulty expressing
emotions in general. She told us that after her husband's
death her zest for life was gone. She became passive and
depressed. Her eating habits also changed: she began to
gulp food down quickly and to overeat. By the time she was
twenty-four she weighed 180 pounds.

Melissa's passivity and her alienation from her own
feelings were reflected in her behavior. She drifted along,
went on welfare, became pregnant again and had an ille-
gitimate child when she was twenty-eight. Three years
later, Melissa married again. She had two more children
before her second husband deserted her. At thirty-three
she felt totally inadequate to care for her four children,
and she began giving them up to foster homes.

The assaults to Melissa's self-esteem over the thirteen
years reported here document her repeated failures to
save herself. When Melissa lost her first husband, her self-
esteem was demolished. If her identity and self-regard
had been strong enough, she could have taken active and
creative direction of her own life. Instead, her opinion of
herself plummeted: she was the widow of a dead criminal;
she was a nobody. Melissa tried to stop feeling, using food
to cushion the pain of her existence. For her next husband
she chose a "worthless" man because she felt unworthy
herself.

Events in her adult life precipitated Melissa's eating
problem, although—as with many adult-onset overeaters
—the roots of her emotional difficulties lay in her own
childhood. Her personality and eating habits had many
traits reminiscent of the anal cluster: low self-esteem,
alienation from feelings, passivity, depression, and gulping of food are all part of the anal character. With stress
she regressed emotionally to that stage.

When Melissa gulped down her food, she was swallowing what the world "dished out," just as children must do

when their mothers force food on them that they do not want. Swallowing the food meant for Melissa that she was going to accept life no matter how bad it was. She didn't chew it well enough to enjoy it, to feel she had assimilated it and made it her own. The food and the layers of fat that followed felt alien to her. She was in a way protecting and isolating the lost, sensitive, younger woman within her, so that the harsh realities of life could not touch what was buried in her distended body. The overeating must also have served as a form of self-punishment for falling into such bad luck.

Another aspect of Melissa's overeating seemed to represent a fusion between mother and child. The death of her first husband tore asunder her newly found adult sense of self and pride. She regressed to where it was safe and protected, to where she hoped to lose her sense of being a "bad" person. By overeating she longed to re-fuse with her mother, with whom she had been very close. Being the only daughter in her family probably also contributed to Melissa's diminished sense of a separate self. When something bad happened to her as a baby, she could cling to her mother. Apparently, food was central to this clinging relationship—a characteristic of the oral-cluster overeater's syndrome. Thus, her overeating was complexly rooted in primitive parts of her personality and served many purposes common to both the oral and anal clusters.

Melissa's adult traumas and problems caused her to regress to these more primitive parts of her personality where overeating was a central defense. To change her lifestyle and repair the damage would require hard work and dedication, plus far better luck than chance and society had provided her with. She was lost and alienated, unable to sustain intimacy in her relationships, isolated within herself. She could not handle the adult stage of generativity, whose primary concern is the guidance of the next generation. Instead, she gave up her children.

JULIE: THE CAREER WOMAN

Adult-onset overeaters are not always victims of misfortune. Sometimes conditions in their lives are very promising, as they were in our next case, the story of a young woman named Julie. Unlike many of her peers, Julie found an answer to the question of her identity rather quickly as an adolescent. Unfortunately, her answer was based almost exclusively on what her parents wanted her to be. Tall, slim, bright, she had been given just enough freedom and opportunity to achieve what her parents expected. Her accomplishments were rewarding: Julie was an honor student at an Ivy League college, and graduated summa cum laude. The marks of achievement were part of her style, part of an identity firmly planted by her family.

Julie was one of two beautiful and intelligent daughters. Her father was a dynamic intellectual role model—full of ideas about spartan mental discipline. Her mother was an austere physical role model—controlled and impeccably organized in appearance and household routine. As for the use of food in this home, it followed a very structured, controlled procedure: Julie's mother gave the two girls and their father each a plate at meal time, brought to the table directly from the kitchen. On each plate was the food she expected them to eat, in exactly the portion she considered adequate. There was never a family-style meal with second helpings or servings from the middle of the table to pass along and choose from.

From this home Julie stepped into the adult world. Having just turned twenty, she found her own apartment and followed her early career plans. As she completed her studies to become an English teacher, she also began courtship and became engaged. She traveled a bit and then got married. Life looked promising, and Julie was looking forward to a future of more creativity and productivity.

But once Julie moved out of her parents' home her eating behavior changed. She went on binges. To keep from gaining too much weight, she then went on crash diets. Overeating was a warning that the controls she had internalized from her parents were not adequate for her as an independent adult. As she overate she rejected parental controls, goals, and expectations. Meals and snacks became a way of procrastinating while she was trying to finish one of her expected tasks. She had chosen to be an English teacher, but when books and papers felt like drudgery to her, she calmed her frustration and confusion by overindulging in cookies and donuts.

When Julie was under stress to produce, she felt tense and anxious. The binges that preceded the meticulous preparations necessary to teaching were a way of postponing the performance her parents were expecting of her. The overeating was her way of rebelling against the job she had to do, a job not freely chosen. She considered the food binges as her own personally chosen rebellions: most of the time she did what was expected of her, yet surreptitiously she took time off every three or four days to fill up on her own choices.

For a few years Julie avoided individual achievements altogether. After her marriage she helped her husband with his career and then became pregnant. In that condition, Julie felt shapeless. The weight that had been creeping up on her over the past few years suddenly zoomed. The doctor was alarmed, and so was Julie. She felt dumpy and the increased weight felt foreign to her. "Who am I now?" her body seemed to be saying. When motherhood came, she still had a confused body-image and a lost personal identity.

Julie took some small jobs while her baby was young, but did not really know what to do with herself. Being an English teacher had felt like drudgery to her, and being a mother seemed no more rewarding. For the next four years she continued, slowly, to gain weight. Julie often

wondered at that time if she should simply stay overweight and get pregnant again. But she kept postponing
that decision too until her child was four. By then she was
so overweight, depressed, and confused that she sought
help with her identity problems.

Julie's identity gave her trouble because of the strong
controls imposed during her childhood. As a little girl, she
had very limited space for experiment and exploration of
her own appetites. Her meals never included choices. She
did not really know what she would put on her own plate
if she were feeding herself. Julie was in her twenties before she tested these controls. When she tried new patterns
of eating, she never knew how far her binges would take
her. How many boxes of cookies could she eat? At home
there had never been any boxes of cookies—just two
vanilla wafers served on a small dish with a large glass of
milk.

When Julie acquired the freedom of managing her own
home for her own family, with her own meals to plan, she
looked for guidelines. As many people do, she fell back
unconsciously on the same controls her mother had used.
She carefully guided her own child's food selection, limit-
ing his choices to what was supposed to be healthy and
sensible. At the same time, she was very perplexed about
the adult choices she had to make for herself: did she want
more children, or a career in teaching, or to become a
writer, or invent a new field that no one had ever expected
or predicted for her? . . .

By her late twenties, Julie had almost eight years and
over forty pounds of confusion weighing upon her. Unable
to get out of her slump of indecision, binges, diets, and
self-doubt, Julie needed help. With professional therapy
she learned to tune into her own hungers and desires, both
for food and for a career. She was able to take deliberate
steps to feed herself in a manner appropriate to what she
really craved, and even learned to let her son find what he

wanted to eat, instead of trying to keep constant control over his appetite, as her mother had done to her.

Julie remembers that her new self-confidence was just beginning to emerge when her son was about five. She had taken him to a dinner buffet and for the first time ever she dared to tell him that he could eat anything he wanted. The little boy began with the main meal and ate moderately. Then he took himself to the dessert table and chose a piece of chocolate cake. When he had eaten it he returned to the dessert table and selected a pudding. But he found that he didn't want to eat all of the pudding and he didn't want to return to try any of the other desserts. Julie, who had projected her own fears of uncontrollable gluttony onto her son, was amazed and fascinated. With external controls removed, she discovered that hunger had its own natural satiation—that genuinely made choices, unlike compulsions, are satisfying.

With objective guidance, Julie was also able to decide on a new profession and started work that felt real to her. She focused and developed her career direction and began to feel as if she knew what she wanted to do and be in her adult life. She found less need to use up time and energy in her vicious cycles of binging and dieting. To some extent, overeating had been her way of acting out the shapelessness she felt when she didn't know what direction she was going in. Without clear goals for her personal performance, she felt blurred and diffuse. As the goals got clearer, and felt like they belonged to her, she procrastinated less in attaining them. She still allowed herself her cravings, but the eating was not a confused compulsion. She discovered tools for adult decision-making that she had not learned as a child. She lost the weight she had gained during the early years of adulthood, just as she gained a true identity separate from parental controls and expections.

For Julie, overeating had been a maladaptive pattern of

behavior, since it did not help her find answers to the questions that plagued her. Choosing to binge on cookies and donuts did not bring her nearer to knowing what choice she wished to make for her own career. Seeking career counseling and professional guidance was adaptive behavior that lead to appropriate adult solutions to her dilemma, even if they came many years and many pounds after her problems first appeared.

SUMMARY

For Millie, overeating had not helped her feel better about the disruption in her sex life. She tried to use food to comfort herself and to hold back her anger, but she continued to feel lonely and deserted. Being overweight simply added to her problems. Her overeating was certainly maladaptive; when sex counseling and some sound scientific information for her husband were introduced, they did indeed offer a solution to Millie's problem.

For Kenneth, adult overeating was related to much earlier conflicts stemming from childhood. When he lost his childhood techniques for coping with problems, his weight went up. He needed to find new, adult solutions to feelings of anger and fear and healthy ways of becoming expressive and independent. Though it was the adult Kenneth who had a weight problem, it was the two-year-old inside him who needed treatment.

Giving nurturance and support as a spouse or parent are adult roles which can trigger childish needs and emotional hungers. In the case of Melissa, adult trauma during her years of marriage and childrearing caused her to regress to the more primitive stage of personality development which uses overeating as a major form of defense against trouble.

Adult-onset overeating is specifically related to latter-day circumstances a person encounters and to the tools he has to handle them. In terms of diagnosis and treatment, the first issue to look at is what is happening in the person's life when overeating begins. Weaknesses from childhood and adolescence appear in maladaptive behavior and inadequate emotional responses. Professional help is usually needed to find the more adaptive behavior and to strengthen the patient's ability to handle the newly arisen problems.

8

---·---

Society and the
Overeater

---·---

*T*hus far in this book we have presented cases and findings which by and large support the contention that overeating is due primarily to emotional problems. These problems are, of course, rooted in the way a person responds to and interacts with the people around him. The individual nurturing figures involved in his upbringing color his responses, but it must be stressed now that society as a whole frequently dictates the quality of these interpersonal relationships, setting the standards by which we live. As we shall see in this chapter, society and its subcultures tend to dictate eating patterns to the family, which in turn greatly influences the child's eating behavior.

FEAST OR FAMINE

One of the basic functions of a society is its ability to make food available to the individual. In middle-class America this function is frequently taken for granted, but for some unfortunate persons the availability of food can never be assumed. In the case of Harry, described in Chapter 3, food was not readily available. Harry's mother withheld both food and love, which formed the basis of his excessive eating in later life when food was abundant. Though Harry had enough food to stay alive and to grow during his childhood, its availability was permeated by the tenuous and hostile aspects of its presentation. These parental responses to him affected Harry's eating patterns for the rest of his life. For him—for every infant—the first crucial social experience is with the person feeding him.

Society's approach to feeding children varies from culture to culture, and from one period of history to another. One concrete example of change is when famine affects a society. Ravelli and his colleagues studied 300,000 men who were exposed to famine in Belgium in 1944–45.[1] The study was made when the men were all nineteen years old and ready to be inducted into the military. Those who had been exposed to the brief famine during the last three months of their mothers' pregnancies and the first months of their lives during the early part of 1944 tended to have few weight problems. Ravelli concluded that because of their nutritional deprivation during this early period of fat cell development, their fat cell number was lower than normal and that when they grew up they had fewer fat cells to feed and so ate less and stayed thinner than normal.

Despite our overall agreement with the fat cell hypothesis (see Chapter 2), we would like to raise the possibility of a far simpler explanation for this documented phenomenon. These army recruits had been born at a time when food was very scarce. Like Harry, they evidently had enough food to stay alive for that year, but conditions of famine meant that the availability of food was extremely tenuous. Unlike Harry, however, love and care was not withheld by their mothers, despite the scarcity of food. Emotional nurturance was given to the Belgian babies, not abundant food. During this critical period of psychological development, these newborns did not experience, in behavioristic terms, the pairing of love and food. When they grew older and experienced other kinds of insecurity and stress, they did not resort to overeating because the availability of food and of love and security had not been linked. These young men were thinner than normal as adults because overeating was not the way they had learned to deal with stress.

The statistics in Ravelli's study reveal too that the babies exposed to the famine during the first half of their mothers' pregnancies tended to have a much higher incidence of obesity than normal. Halfway through their mothers' pregnancies, the famine ended; these babies were born when food was again available. It seems to us, therefore, that the fat cell theory cannot explain why these later babies have a higher incidence of obesity. Ravelli evoked the hypothesis that this prenatal nutritional deprivation may have affected the appetite centers in the hypothalami of the fetuses. However, society too had experienced a trauma that must certainly have changed the mothers' attitudes toward provisions. Frightened by famine during pregnancy, these mothers did link food and security; food became readily available after having been so dear. For these mothers food and love must have been more closely linked than normal, and it seems quite likely that they would impart this feeling to their infants. As children and young adults, then, these men might readily have resorted to eating in times of stress and show a higher incidence of obesity than normal, as the data indicated.

A parallel phenomenon may have occurred in middle-class American culture during the Depression years, when food was not readily obtainable. Attitudes concerning food and security were certainly affected by this experience. Food was dear, though not as scarce as during the famine in Belgium. However, the real possibility exists that many American mothers reacted somewhat like the mothers after the Belgian famine when food became readily available again: these mothers probably paired food with closeness, warmth, love, and security. Their children would sense this attitude and in later times of isolation and stress would tend to look for comfort in eating. One would predict, therefore, more overeating and a higher incidence of obesity than normal in post-Depression babies. These post-Depression attitudes about eating probably affected future generations of Americans.

Other changes in food consumption that occurred after the Depression still pervade our society. Infants tended to be given the bottle in addition to or instead of being breast-fed. They also tended to be fed solid foods earlier. This meant that everyone in the family, not only the mother, could participate in feeding the baby—grandparents, sisters, brothers, fathers, and other relatives. These formerly peripheral persons were no longer restricted to playing with and cuddling the baby; now they were able to feed it. Since more people could interact with the newborn by offering the bottle or solid food, if the baby ate well for any particular person, it was taken as a sign that the child liked him or her best.

The pairing of eating and emotional closeness thus became even stronger and more pervasive because the eating experience itself now became a part of several important relationships in the child's life. As emphasized in earlier chapters, problems with fusion are frequently at the root of an overeating problem. The link between eating, emotional closeness, and security is almost indelible. When linked excessively, the long-term results can also be excessive.

Other characteristics of American society appear to reinforce the link between food and closeness. It is part of our society to connect good food with good times. It is not simply that all forms of advertisements stress food—radio, TV, magazines, and newspapers—but that they link food with family togetherness, with women pleasing men, men courting women, mothers showing love and care, grand-mas providing high-calorie treats. To sell food, commercials play upon our society's hunger for love and security. Unfortunately, the people who are most easily influenced by this kind of advertising are those with the deeper emotional hungers. Persons who are able to resist the lure of the commercials are generally those healthier members of society whose emotional hungers are being satisfied in other ways.

Most of this book is about the grown-up children who have emotional hungers. If they can understand what it is they really hunger for—meaningful and fulfilling human relationships—they might stop trying to fill the hunger by overeating. This requires tuning into the self instead of into the incessant stimuli provided by advertisements. Frequently people need professional help to acquire the insights necessary to an understanding of themselves. It also requires strength of will to act on this new understanding, and it takes courage to reach out to others to have one's emotional needs met. It takes little strength or courage to pull open the refrigerator door.

Inner strength is difficult to achieve, since all the stages of childhood development leave us with scars and weaknesses that can affect our eating behavior. In addition, there is an insidious external force that needs to be combated: the diet food industry, in which are included advertising, production, and distribution of diet aids, drugs, sugar-free drinks, low-calorie foods, diet books, and reducing clinics. All are proliferating in today's economy, along with the advertisement, production, and distribution of cheap, fast, fattening foods and drinks and the restaurants in which these are sold. A society of overeaters and compulsive dieters maintains this very busy industry, which holds out the promise of easy, instant cures for obesity. Since obese people are more sensitive to external cues than non-obese people, they respond more to today's food advertising. Our society has created a constant crisis for them and increased their vulnerability to tempting oral stimuli.

Erik Erikson, in *Childhood and Society,* suggests that a society's culture provides certain balances in later life for the very desires, fears, and rages that the cultural conditioning provokes in childhood.[2] It is possible that in our culture we rear babies who need to eat, eat, eat, quick, quick, quick. Demand feedings, for example, has been popular in America for several decades: an infant is fed when it cries. In hospital maternity wards, in the first days of life, the practice is to give sugar water to babies when they cry between feedings. Later, mothers offer pacifiers or extra bottles of juice or milk. This practice is continued when whining or fretful toddlers are given a cracker or cookie to quiet them or to reward them when they are cooperative.

This cultural characteristic of instant gratification permeates American society today: a flick of the switch gives us immediate entertainment on television or radio. Charge accounts and bank loans increase our spending power much faster than would building up a savings account by dint of patience and thrifty habits. We have quick-drying paints for our homes, fast-food services for our meals, instantaneous-cooking ovens for our kitchens, super-powered dryers for our hair. Encounter groups and mating services provide people with quick intimacy and instant friends. We need never wait for our vegetables to grow or even to come into season, since all varieties of fruits and vegetables are found in stores, frozen or shipped fresh across the country. Very few people any longer connect having meats with the long and patient vigil of primitive man's hunting expeditions—and with reason, since poultry and livestock are fattened up and injected with chemicals to bring them to the slaughterhouses and our tables in record time.

These conditions of technological society are particularly pertinent to people with eating problems. Since many obese people have had trouble in early stages of ego development, their resulting immature personalities require immediate gratification. The obese have difficulty postponing their rewards and seek comfort from whatever is most easily obtainable. The food industry in our society makes certain that treats are readily available at prices most people can afford, and in so doing perpetuates the problem of obesity.

THE COMMUNITY

Culture influences every aspect of eating—not only what foods are considered desirable, but what times of the day or night to eat, in whose company, in what position, and for what purpose. According to the culture of any given society, the purpose of eating may be primarily for bodily sustenance; for the sake of virtue or pleasure; or for social or religious communion. In a melting-pot society such as we have in America, various subcultures have their own eating traditions that have been transported from the Old World. The more functions a particular subculture assigns to its eating experience, the more important food itself seems to be to the people raised within those cultural influences.

Some subcultures assign more importance to the eating experience than others. This is verified in medical literature reporting on the socio-economic, ethnic, and religious variables related to the incidence of obesity.[3,4,5] Among Jews, Latins, and Middle Europeans, the eating experience is likely to serve many special purposes: meals are social times for underscoring the value of warm family life. These gatherings are a time to eat out of respect and honor for the person who has prepared the meal. Eating well is a virtue and a duty—a symbol of being obedient, cooperative, and accepting. Extra weight on children in these ethnic groups is frequently considered a preventive health measure, or even a sign of the family's financial prosperity. The gatherings are sometimes religious observances as well, beginning and ending in prayers or blessings, with traditional foods designated for specific religious occasions.

Close-knit, traditional-minded subcultures seem to link maternal love and nurturance with food, and there appears at first glance to be a higher incidence of obesity among such groups as well, although rigorous scientific documentation is lacking. Investigations made to date do, however, relate social factors—including class and religion—to whether a person will have weight problems in life. The implications are that the individual's psychodynamics concerning food definitely need to be viewed in light of cultural traditions and attitudes.

When the dinner table is a central family arena, the eating experience gathers significance. The event is not simply meant to fill one's stomach. To eat together is to relate, laugh, joke, argue, tease, discuss the world's affairs or their own. Gathered together for these events, families share food and intimacy. Eating thus becomes a communion or a social fusion.[6] When the children of these families venture into the "outside" world, they may yearn, especially during times of stress, for the closeness, support, and sense of communion they remember inside the family. During these times people need strength: some look to God for help (they can even fuse, in a sense, with God by means of a religious communion), others long for closeness and communion with family, which seemed almost an omnipotent source of strength during their early childhood. The family, however, may not be as accessible or available as it once was, or the young person may be trying to be independent and to avoid family support. Therefore fusion is attempted through compulsive overeating, which had been so strongly paired with closeness in childhood.

To treat overeating with success, the various emotional values of food have to be considered, as well as such cultural factors as the symbolic values subcultures or the extended family place on the eating experience. An effective diet must provide these symbolic values in other ways: the overeater needs to find other ways of feeling dutiful or virtuous or religious or loyal. If food has been a symbol of acceptance or security, other offerings of acceptance or security must be provided to nourish the soul while the body diets.

Momism

Various subcultures have been assimilated into American society in recent decades, and in this process of transplanting and rerooting a lifestyle and a set of values has developed that we will refer to as Momism. It is predicated on the assumption that a "good" mother is one who gives totally to her children, not only during the early years to assure her infants' survival, but throughout the prolonged childhood, adolescence, and even adulthood of her offspring.

Momism is a system that proclaims that children come first. Mom's primary goal is to be the feeder and giver, responsible for preparing and offering the food. This role is extended to many aspects of the eating experience. Extended nurturance becomes the hallmark of her existence.

Momism became quite pervasive in American culture as the ethnic subcultures intermingled and blended into the society. Only with the onset of the feminist movement and the growing trend of women to hold jobs outside the home has Momism decreased its stranglehold on a generation or more of American families.

The effects of Momism involve a curious combination of psychodynamics and sociodynamic factors whose influence on children warrants inspection. Mom, powerful in her dedication to nurturing, became terribly important to her children's existence, and they to hers. She needed to cultivate her children's dependency on her, for if they were to break free they would desert her and deny her reason for existing. Growing away from Mom—a healthy and natural developmental step—is then associated with guilt, shame, and ambivalence, not growth and development. The children of such women have a great deal of difficulty exerting their own independence and initiative, and have only a nebulous notion of their separate identities.

As we stated in our discussion of the anal cluster, problems of independence are key issues for many overeaters, especially the anal types, who constitute the largest group of overeaters. Children raised in the shadow of Momism often experience the urge to fuse as an alternative to independence. Since eating in their families had been a warm and close family event orchestrated by Mom, food becomes a solution to stress during times that require initiative and independent action. Overeating is the symbolic expression of the ambivalence concerning initiative. Momism, which fostered a need to fuse, now appears to be a common factor in many anal-cluster overeaters.

Daughters of these Moms did not see in their mothers the pursuit of any major source of gratification outside of mothering itself. Lee, the daughter of one such woman, was discussed in detail in Chapter 5. Lee's background was of Polish-Russian extraction. She was a very bright little girl who quickly learned to copy her mother. She played with dolls and, like many little girls, her chief activity was feeding and dressing them. Later, when her baby sister was born, she transferred this make-believe mothering onto this live "doll." It happened that Lee's feeding and caring for her baby sister were reinforced by her environment, while her participation in other activities was virtually disregarded. The praise and attention that she got for being the good older sister far outweighed support for any of her other achievements. Lee was deeply gratified by being considered a good giver, just as her family was deeply pleased by her helping her mother.

As a child Lee embraced Momism, since giving to people who needed her was the thing that worked best for her survival. She became a school teacher, which enabled her to keep giving. She married a man who needed a Mom, which perpetuated this role. And, finally, she had a baby —the giving role par excellence.

Since Momism was her predestined role, Lee's child became her main object of nurturance. This upset her relationship with her husband because their marriage had been based on her giving him the nurturance he needed. He felt terribly deprived when their baby arrived, and left his wife. This meant that Lee had only one form of gratification remaining: giving to her children. With no close relationship left between herself and her husband, there was little hope of receiving some adult form of gratification. No one was giving to her; no one was feeding her in terms of food or love or support. Her own needs became starved for attention, starved for their own satisfaction and gratification.

But Lee knew only one way for a woman to gratify her needs—through nurturance. She felt her own neediness keenly, but the only act she could ever accomplish to fill these needs was to feed herself. She returned to the form of gratification that her Mom had taught her, and secretly fed her hungry self. Her secret was betrayed as the years went by: Lee became quite overweight.

Dolly, described in Chapter 3, grew up in an Italian home. Her mother also epitomized Momism. Her particular background was especially geared to and adept at fusing the generations. As young people grow up in such an atmosphere, they continue to look for some way of reenacting the emotional fusion they experienced in childhood. They may establish a very consuming relationship with a spouse who will act as a lover and a nurturer, filling their emotional needs. Some establish a close-knit family of their own when they marry so that they can partially satisfy their need to fuse again. Their prognosis is not always bad; some of them can in fact lead successful and fulfilling lives. Involvement in religion and mysticism are two ways in which the self may partially merge into a larger whole without resorting to unhealthy patterns of eating.

The mother-child relationship that incorporates excessive nurturing gets perpetuated as new families are created in the image of old ones. The great, giving Mom feels she is "sacrificing all for her children, yet by feeling this she actually fuses with them and renders them overly dependent on her. However, at the root of her giving is a real neediness, a real emptiness. She *needs* to fuse, as did her own mother." She cannot truly stand on her own two feet. Erikson characterizes such a woman as "vain . . . , egotistical . . . , and infantile."[7] She is not someone who can be relied on and, therefore, she will ultimately let her children down. They were promised nurturance and an all-giving mother; instead, as they get older, they discover her to be a basically weak woman who cannot provide for herself, let alone her children. She needs them to try and make herself whole.

Of course, many a mother who appears supportive and giving does have genuinely adequate resources of her own and a true ability to give. She has developed a strong identity, trusts in herself, finds her own life meaningful, and has no need to fuse excessively with her children. This woman is not a representative of Momism. Her children can develop a sense of independence and security, since their appetite for closeness and fusion has been adequately filled by a mother who could nourish them emotionally. Mother did not drain them of their inner strength; therefore, they are not left with a compulsive hunger.

Interestingly, anorexia nervosa appears to be more common in families with Moms. When young girls, typically sixteen to twenty-two years of age, develop this disease, the causes are considered psychological. These are girls who have reached a stage in life of conflict around issues of sexuality—menstruation, dating, marriage, etc. They are anxious about their femininity, and they are not getting along with their domineering mothers. The daughters' attempt to break away from these Moms is a rebellion which is peculiarly symbolic and yet concrete. Mother, the dominant nurturer, is a symbol of food and of female sexuality. Anorexic girls, therefore, reject food to the point of emaciation or death and also concrete aspects of their sexuality, such as curved hips and breasts.[8] They do not seem able to break away from their powerful mothers in an adult-like fashion.

A SELF-FULFILLING PROPHECY: THE CASE OF MICHELLE

The psyche of a parent and the atmosphere of the family are obviously the first social factors to affect the child's eating pattern. The emotional environment the parents create affects how the child feels about itself, how satisfied or hungry it is emotionally. The physical environment the parents provide can make a difference in the availability of the "right" or "wrong" foods. Just as important, with the birth of a child comes a new set of hopes, anticipations, and expectations. The mother and father place their beliefs about themselves as adults and parents into what they believe to be true about their child. Much of what they expect from their children comes from what they know of themselves.

It has been noted that a parent frequently picks one child to identify with more than any of the other children a couple may have. The mother may choose her first-born daughter, the father his first-born son. But this is by no means the rule. Other patterns occur; for example, a mother who was a middle child may choose her own middle child to favor, be it a boy or a girl.

We see, then, two general ways that parents relate to their children. One is the overall set of expectations they have for their whole family, the other is the close identity they form when they see a particular part of themselves reflected in an individual child. A resulting phenomenon is that the parent has a feeling or belief about that child's future which is really based primarily on what has happened or what he wanted to happen in his own life. Out of these feelings and beliefs he constructs a kind of prophecy about how the child will develop, and often that prophecy becomes self-fulfilling.[9]

The preconceived ideas parents have about what the future holds for their children can cover many subjects. For instance, a mother or father may have felt that the world was a very dangerous place for them and will transmit that attitude to their children. A parent may have found that being intimate with people of the opposite sex produced painful experiences for them, and so will pass this message on to the child. The parent may have grown up feeling awkward and clumsy or graceful and attractive, and may expect that their child will feel similarly.

Examples of how the self-fulfilling prophecy works can be seen throughout a child's life. An earnest mother registers her young daughter for dancing classes. On the first day of class she goes in with her child to meet the teacher and explains that she, the mother, has always been so clumsy that she wants her daughter to grow up with more grace and for that reason is starting her in dancing school. How different that message is from that of another mother who announces that ever since she was very little she loved dancing and wants her little girl to have a chance to enjoy it too.

Many of the messages that children pick up from their parents are indirect messages. Parents who feel, for example, that bad luck always plagues them can give their children the feeling that the world is unlucky without ever saying so in just so many words. Children are susceptible to these messages because they identify with the parents.

In later life, when the child begins to get feedback from the rest of the world, no message has the impact of these early communications.

Applying this basic principle to the subject of eating patterns and body-image seems relevant: the parent who finds that food is one of his or her main sources of pleasure cannot help but feel that what the child has to eat will be its source of pleasure. If the parent does not have any other major source of pleasure, how is he or she going to give the child other values or ideas about where to get pleasurable experiences? The child who sees a parent constantly torn by temptations of overeating and who sees himself as an extension of that parent will naturally adopt the same feelings about food. If a child sees that a parent eats when he is bored, or angry, or happy, or nervous, or tired, or socially engaged, or sexually excited (yes, children *can* sense all these feelings going on around them), then eating begins to serve that function for him, too. Obesity may run in families, not so much because it runs in the hereditary genes of that family, but because it is ingrained in its food habits and food values.[10] It runs in the social structure of the family, between parent and child: "I'm fat, you'll be fat"; "You're fat, I'm going to be fat." Sometimes it is unspoken, but always the expectations are there, fostering the self-fulfilling images.

For a beautiful young lady named Michelle, one powerful prophecy operated: eat and you will be happy. With a radiant and dimpled smile on her face, she struggled continually with her weight. It was terribly important to Michelle that she eat well and look well, since the single and sustained message she had received from her parents was that she was pretty and if she always smiled and stayed healthy, everything would be all right. Overprotected and overfed, Michelle weighed 147 pounds by the time she was fourteen. Being "sweet" meant eating the abundant Italian specialties prepared by her mother.

Michelle's parents never suggested that she develop hobbies and skills or pursue an education or career. They assured her that she was pretty enough not to have to worry about any of that. They gave her no alternative ways of coping with her future other than being pretty and healthy. It appears that Michelle's health and appearance were even more crucial to her parents because her mother suffered from multiple sclerosis. Michelle was an only child, born late in her mother's life, and simply by staying healthy and looking beautiful she was adored; little else was asked of her. She grew up in an apartment in a neighborhood without peers, and had few friends to demand more from her. This isolation further ensured that no other more helpful messages about how she might cope would reach her.

Well-functioning role models were very limited in Michelle's world. Because of her mother's chronic illness, Michelle did not have a coping woman to identify with. Her mother's major accomplishment—which took a great deal of effort—was to be able to function well enough within the home to provide some of the traditional Italian dishes for her family. The prime challenge for most little girls, to win daddy from mommy, required no effort at all: to be daddy's girl, Michelle had only to stay pretty and not get hurt or sick. For most of her childhood Michelle even shared her parents' bedroom.

Michelle met all anxious situations by one method alone: smiling, sitting very still, poised, her imperturbable beauty her only defense against tension, anger, attack, or loss. She had internalized the family edict to smile and be healthy and everything will be all right. When she was insulted she smiled—an amazing thing to behold. She did not return with a cutting remark of her own, having been taught never to risk aggressive behavior for fear she might be hurt. The chubby little Michelle was praised also for her quietness, never running or romping about. As a grown woman, she maintained her superficial smile, learned to cook as well as her mother, and quietly watched her dimples spread.

Parents, relatives, friends all tell children what they think the young person is able to do well, often with the well-meaning intention of bolstering their self-confidence. Some of these messages become self-fulfilling prophecies: when the child constantly hears that he is good at something in particular, confidence develops in that area. These prophecies become even more important during stressful situations. For example, if the parents have instilled in the child the message that he is good with his hands, or has a talent for woodwork, the grown-up child may find himself in his basement one day making bookends as his business collapses. The woodwork in the basement is a kind of security blanket that lets him feel momentarily skillful, safe, and coping creatively with life. The defensive behavior becomes repetitive and habitual only if other forms of behavior that offer a sense of competence have never been reinforced.

How does such a system of negative messages develop? Overprotective parents may prevent their child's exposure to a wider variety of messages of competence, urging the child to come to mommy and daddy when there is a problem or a question. In this case the underlying message is that the child cannot handle the problem alone. Most children learn to identify with their overprotective parents and so internalize their problem-solving ability. Thus they feel they have acquired their parents' competence and are able to avoid undue difficulties. However, in a few instances, such as the case of Michelle, identification with a model who has poor ways of coping may result in very limited coping mechanisms for the child.

Being a "good" eater is a common message of competence. Eating is one of the earliest forms of behavior, and so parents are particularly attuned to it. Parents are eager to attach such character traits to their child so that the infant does not remain an anonymous being. Interestingly, good eaters tend to be happy, smiling babies. Colicky babies have trouble eating and tend to cry a good deal. Good eaters are not only given the message that they are good eaters, but along with it the message that they are happy-go-lucky. This prophecy can become self-fulfilling, for they may indeed become happy-go-lucky, overweight adults. When later external suggestions are made that they diet for health and slimness, the prospect seems overwhelmingly unhappy.

If an overeater has a basic self-image that links being a good eater with being a happy-go-lucky person, dieting must be approached with caution. Losses of food for the sake of diet may be interpreted as losses of goodness and happiness. This points out once again that before dieting can be successful, it is essential to explore the meaning of food to the individual, its meaning in the family, and its meaning to the existing self-image. In order to understand this crucial area, the overeater must tune in to his early experiences with his parents, their prejudices and expectations. He can then become more aware of how his image of himself is related to what he eats. Certain important foods that symbolize an image, such as the happiness of childhood that an overeater may be trying to hold onto, should probably be incorporated into the diet if it is to be successful. Michelle offers an excellent example of that: she learned to diet by restricting her carbohydrate intake to warm, crusty Italian bread. She gave up cream sauces but allowed herself thick Italian tomato sauces. The bread was her link to dimpled girlhood and the tomato sauce was her way of appreciating her mother's efforts. These emotionally important calories were included in her otherwise lean diet.

Michelle came to understand herself well enough to nurture herself in non-oral ways—a key to successful dieting. She learned to reinterpret the message to look pretty and stay healthy by preoccupying herself with clothes, suntan lotions, and beauty creams. She overinvested in vitamin pills. Through all these activities, she felt she was staying pretty and healthy—and she also found she was staying slim. These substitutes became her new symbols of health and beauty.

HOW WE FEED OUR CHILDREN

Parental messages are one of the social factors that govern eating habits. Another is the society's feeding practices. Does the society feed its children when they demand it or according to a strict schedule? American society is a great melting pot of child-feeding techniques, since various subcultures feed their children in differing ways. In recent years our overall child-feeding practice has undergone a drastic change that is in harmony with some of the other technical changes we have experienced. Whereas in the 1940s strict feeding schedules for infants were the rule, since the late 1950s demand feeding has been the vogue. These changes have created new stresses for some members of our society.

The child fed according to a time schedule eventually learns to expect food at specific intervals; the child learns to rely on the external environment to tell him when to eat. The social system structures these needs and expectations, then satisfies them. Thus the need for food becomes a part of the child's socialization process. Unlike the schedule-fed child, the demand-fed baby eats according to its inner pangs of hunger, not as the result of an externally imposed schedule. It has the opportunity in its early childhood to develop a refined awareness of hunger as felt in its own body.

Children who were schedule-fed have an advantage in some social circumstances. For example, young people in such social institutions as camps or boarding schools were very comfortable up to the mid-1960s. They were expected to conform to the structure of the institution, which was highly regulated. For the most part, eating took place at eight, noon, and six. Alternatives were not available. Perhaps a canteen selling food was open at a specific afternoon or evening hour, but these were never extravagant. Since these school children had been brought up to fit into this regime, schedule-feeding seemed natural. As infants, each child had learned to trust the environment, and indeed it lived up to his expectations. His society was happily consistent with his upbringing.

However, times have changed. The children who were raised on demand-feeding are now having a growing influence on American society. Our culture is providing less of the institutions and the environment for eating behavior that fits the character of the person raised on schedule feeding. Students demand food machines so that they can have snacks at any time. In many homes children tend to have free access to the refrigerator. Because they are sensitive to their inner need for food, they do not depend on external guides to tell them how much and when to eat. It is natural for them to listen to their own cravings, since they do not eat compulsively. Young people born in the 1950s are the ones who now flock to fast-food restaurants. They demand their food now and they want to eat it now. Society has changed to reflect the character of these new adults, as witnessed by the proliferation of prepackaged meals and fast-food chains.

The adult who in childhood was schedule-fed has not been prepared for this new change in society. He cannot cope with the over-availability and over-abundance of food. He could trust his environment when it told him what he needed and when. He therefore did not develop a strong sensitivity to his inner need for food. In today's fast-food culture he has trouble passing up a candy machine with all those appealing, colorful wrappers. A snack bar that is always open, a grocery that sells food twenty-four hours a day, fast foods at every corner—these stimuli confuse him. He does not know how and when to eat in this new society, being overly sensitive to the onslaught of external cues. He tends to be the overeating type in today's Demand Culture.

How We View Obesity

Our attitudes concerning obesity are formed by our culture. These attitudes are quite negative. A slender figure is considered desirable in women, but this attitude is a prejudice created by our society. In other cultures where a value is set on the "pleasantly plump" female figure, young women may stuff themselves in order to achieve that society's ideal. Beauty may be in the eyes of the beholder, but the eyes of the beholder are, in part, a conditioned reflection of the culture at large.

Why does our culture view obesity with disfavor? The value we place on work and productivity may be at the heart of this prejudice. Throughout our literature we hear of the fat, lazy person as if being fat and lazy were synonymous. This stereotype may have arisen because it is thought that if a person is obese he will have difficulty simply moving around, much less working. By contrast, leanness appears to be connected with aggressiveness, quick, decisive action, and hard work. The ambitious, plotting Cassius in Shakespeare's *Julius Caesar* had a "lean and hungry look."

In certain societies excess fat is equated with conspicuous consumption and prosperity. In societies where all food is hard to obtain, the condition of plumpness is only affordable by the wealthy. Husbands are proud that they can keep their wives and children fat. Obesity thus becomes a status symbol.

Various studies have shown a definite relationship between socio-economic class and obesity. Goldblatt et al., for example, have shown (see note 4) that obesity is "six times more common among women of low status as compared to those of high status. More than that, parental status was nearly as important in determining obesity." This suggests that poverty is not only linked with obesity but is a causal factor. Furthermore, the studies of Stunkard et al.[11] seem to show that "obesity is not only more prevalent among poor girls, but this prevalence is established earlier and increases at a more rapid rate than among upper-class girls." By the age of six, obesity was nine times as prevalent in lower-glass girls than their upper-class counterparts.

Because overweight is viewed negatively in our slim-minded society, people with weight problems are not likely to think well of themselves. Therefore, they may expect less for themselves and may settle for less: less in a job, less in marriage, less in their living conditions. These low expectations can be passed from one generation to another in a family in much the same way that unhealthy eating patterns are transmitted. Subcultures, often excluded from the mainstream of upper-class wealth, frequently have family traditions and characteristics which actively promote the development of obesity.[12] Whenever there is a connection between food and family or religious communion, and strong Momism, overeating is more prevalent.

WHAT WE CAN DO

Specifically, steps must be taken to separate food from emotional development, disentangle it from issues of loyalty, guilt, and independence. Not only family communion but religious communion needs to be disassociated from the eating experience. Family get-togethers linked with religious holidays need to move away from the dinner table. Social experiences do not have to be made into food experiences. In spite of instant formulas, babies should not be fed by all the family. The child needs to relate to its family through its eyes, ears, and touch—not simply through its mouth. Parents who have struggled themselves with overeating and overweight need not burden their children with self-fulfilling prophecies of continued overeating problems. The diminishing existence of Momism in our society may help in the future. Certainly, families that can avoid this syndrome have a better chance of avoiding overeating.

In today's Demand Culture feeding infants according to a rigid schedule could be detrimental to their later adjustment, since as the society now exists, demand-fed children do have an advantage. They are part of a society that allows them to demand what and when they wish to eat. If concerned adults can be flexible enough to adjust to these social changes, overeating may be less prevalent in future generations.

9

Movement As Therapy

THE INSTRUMENT: THE BODY

*P*osture, gestures, and habits of moving reveal many of the unspoken—or unspeakable—messages people are transmitting. Since physical movement is both a release of tension and a form of communication, the movement therapies can be used to encourage the body itself to express feelings and fill needs. Dancers develop into an art form the use of body movements to communicate, while many non-performers let their bodies move spontaneously, in daily communication. Unfortunately, many inhibited people cannot move their bodies with ease, and communicate their thoughts and feelings with only the smallest motions.

To whatever degree it is used, it is undeniable that the body is an instrument of expression, and an important tool of communication. Every living body is always moving; strong movements are a sign of health and aliveness. Society dictates that we control some of the ways in which we move, and building those controls is part of normal growth and development, along with expanding our repertoire of movement skills. A child in the womb, if it is growing normally, will kick and move, sometimes quite vigorously. Once born, the baby moves continuously. Physiologically, it is imperative to the infant's growth that he stretch, wiggle, grasp, suck, and make the swimming movements that exercise his limbs.

Body movement is part of human development at every stage of the life cycle. The heart and lungs, for example, are always moving in us involuntarily. Our muscles relax and contract unconsciously. When we sleep our bodies continue to move, not just in the passive rhythms of the metabolic system, but in changes of position and expressions of dreams. When we awake, the passive, mechanical beat inside of us continues. The more actively we exert ourselves, the more we heighten that beat. Our hearts pound and we breathe deeply, increasing our awareness of the mechanical parts of the body. This exertion is physically healthy for the cardiovascular system and psychologically healthy for the sense of a heightened life, the exhilaration of being alive. When we exert ourselves and feel the pulse increase inside us, we are more aware of the life of our own bodies.

Movement is a needed therapeutic antidote to the problems of being alive in the 20th century. Our technological environment differs vastly from the natural one our early ancestors knew. Today we have decreased possibilities for movement: work is being automated, transportation is by wheels, and the energy for turning the wheels usually comes from an engine, not from our arms and legs. Furthermore, and equally significant, "civilized" people do not run, jump, rage, or rejoice in an overly boisterous manner. We are taught, as we are socialized, to control strong feelings and impulses instead of acting them out. The impetuous parts of human nature are brought under control for the sake of social living.

In the specific expressive therapy called dance-movement therapy, a time and place are set aside to allow increased possibilities for movement. The energy that comes from emotions, the agitation, nervousness, restlessness, or excitement that comes with strong feelings, is used in exercise and expression. Movement is encouraged and enlarged so that its meaning may be understood. Since many people are afraid of emotional energy, when they feel anxiety they may overeat as a tranquilizer. The changes in blood sugar slow the body down and reduce the feeling of anxiety. Others try to use up that energy by compulsive cooking, cleaning, or working. Even exercise can be used compulsively to avoid dealing with troublesome issues. The goal is to get rid of the energy by overeating or overdoing, by falling asleep or falling into exhaustion.

In movement therapy, instead of nervous, compulsive expenditure of energy in an avoidance activity, patients are helped to recognize and understand the feelings masked by their activity. The therapist provides some safety and assistance in dealing with feelings that may be painful, frightening, sad, or exciting. Normally, tension is discharged in constructive or recreational activities, but with persons overwhelmed by chronic tensions, pleasurable outlets are often blocked. Therefore, it is important to learn what feelings are being hidden behind the tension.

Compulsive activity is a misuse of energy because it blunts awareness of feelings. Procrastinating rituals frequently involve compulsive patterns of activity, as in the case of the person who must get to work but keeps sharpening pencils before sitting at his desk. Julie, in Chapter 7, prepared elaborate snacks as a way of postponing her desk work. Jack, in Chapter 4, went running for six to eight miles a day. He managed to keep his 200-pound-body in good condition for several years while he postponed examining his extra weight and the nervous tension he was experiencing. Marie, in Chapter 4, once wrote that she often walked out of her house in the middle of an eating binge and went to a bowling alley. She found it easier to force herself to bowl than to force herself to examine her craving for food. These compulsive activities mobilize emotional energy that has been repressed and succeed temporarily in allowing some part of that tension to be discharged.

The connection between physical and emotional tension is always an underlying factor in psychosomatic problems. Overeating, as we have been stressing throughout, is usually a psychosomatic problem. An attitude or feeling, alive in the unconscious, causes some bizarre eating behavior, which in turn causes somatic changes—bloatedness, sluggishness, and obesity.

The physical characteristics of a person's tension (breathing habits among them) are like clues pointing to the mental tensions.[1] The body needs to discharge tension, and an adequate discharge may disturb its chemistry. The warded-off and pent-up instincts and impulses of the unsatisfied person seek substitute outlets, including eating. But substitute outlets are still not sufficient, and a residual amount of tension remains in the body.

This stored tension is like a heavy burden or weight the body carries. Such a condition can be exhausting, and can result in a depression of spirit or energy. The depression may signify the recurrent failure to find satisfactory ways of releasing tension, while the weariness is a result of the amount of energy being used, unconsciously, to keep the troublesome feelings in check. Sometimes the repression is holding back tremendous forces of rage, sometimes strong instinctual sexual drives. The pent-up emotions may involve childhood fears that once seemed too terrifying to face.

The result of chronic tension is frequently seen in the rigidity of various body parts, which have in a sense absorbed all the blocked desires or impulses. A person in movement therapy is first given time to establish a basic trust in the therapeutic setting.[2] He needs to know he is in a reliable, professional, and sensitive relationship and that he will neither hurt the therapist nor himself. Under these safe conditions he is frequently able to use the energy locked in his torso, back, neck, belly, arms, or legs, to break the repression there, and so let the energy flow. With the release of psychogenic tension there is often a feeling of exhilaration.

THE WAY IT WORKED FOR OLGA AND MARTIN

Olga, discussed in Chapter 4, had arms and legs so stiff and rigid that they seemed hardly alive. But she had a difficult time allowing herself to move in a way which would release that rigidity. She was asked to begin by flicking her wrists, as if she had just washed her hands but didn't have a towel. Then she tried flicking from her elbows, and later from her shoulders. Having done this, Olga seemed to have verified for herself that the space she flung her arms into was safe, that no dangers resulted from using that space. This allowed her to make further use of her hands and arms to slash, then pound, the space around her. First her movement was in her wrists, then she slashed from her elbows, and finally took full swings from her shoulders. Olga did not know when she began movement therapy what specific mental tension was causatively associated with her physical tension, and neither did her therapist. But she was able to discharge some of that tension and she was able to feel the exhilaration of the release.

Martin, also described in Chapter 4, had legs that were tight and stiff. The tightness in this musculature was actually causing chronic back pain. Martin needed to release his unconscious inhibitions and anger, and began by doing small heel and toe movements. First he pressed into the floor with each heel. Then he pressed with the ball of each foot, as if he were putting out a cigarette butt. He found he could press as hard as he wanted, with all his strength, and that the floor did not give way. This crushing exercise is intended to provoke anal rage and sadism—taboo feelings for this patient. Martin's stored-up energy felt a release, and a smile appeared on his face. Color rose to his cheeks, his eyes flashed as the energy flowed upward from his feet. He could express his full anger—and still nothing terrifying happened. Martin did exercises to loosen his ankles and kick with his knees, eventually he discovered he could stomp and kick by using his whole leg. It had been proven to him that the world around him was able to absorb and endure his pent-up energy and anger without being harmed, and therefore his body could finally discharge that tension.

When these sessions were over Martin's legs usually trembled and felt loose. He was able to relax; indeed, he deserved to—he had discovered an exercise for his body which was very hard work. The years of holding back had made these movements terribly difficult for him, yet he had triumphed over great odds. His therapeutic achievement left him as relaxed and happy as a good bowel movement might leave a constipated person.

Muscle tightness can cause chronic problems in many different parts of the body. When it is located in the neck, stiffness and headaches can follow. In such cases, the body is perhaps trying to block certain information, emotions, or instincts from rising up to the cognitive level. The first exercises to try for release of neck tension are loud counting and shouting to match simple, nonthreatening movements. For lower back or pelvic area tightness, therapeutic movement includes stretching the lower back area and releasing the blocked energy in that part of the body. When shoulders are tense, appropriate exercises are used to afford release and help the person get the "weight of the world" off his shoulders.

Movement therapy works especially well for those people who have difficulty verbalizing or conceptualizing their problems. Their tension is locked into their bodies, and often overeating is the only behavior they know for trying to cope. A dance or movement therapist tries to help disentangle feelings and find new forms of behavior, not by delving through the mind or intellect, but by addressing himself to the body.

So often the conscious mind does not give permission to the unconscious to verbalize anxious feelings. Intellectual attempts to connect with the unconscious thought are blocked or censored. The body, however, is closer to the unconscious part of the person than words or intellect can ever be. In the case of obesity, the body has in fact already responded visibly by overeating behavior. On some gut level, the body already knows about the problem. But unless it is released, the problem stays at the gut level while the mouth busily keeps undesirable information out of conscious thought.

ACTION IN THE TREATMENT OF MILLIE, ELLEN, RENA, AND ROGER

Millie, the overeater described in Chapter 7 whose husband had stopped having intercourse with her, usually did most of her snacking in the evenings—the times she felt sadness in the pit of her stomach and anger in the form of a feeling of tightness in her chest. Her overeating pattern used food to push these feelings of sadness, loss, and frustration down into her body, out of her head. Millie made no conscious mental efforts to deal with her sexual frustration.

When Millie's physician took her personal history, he was able to identify the events that had affected her eating habits. That overeating had begun when sexual intercourse had stopped was clear from the history. This diagnosis was possible because Millie was herself able to provide the relevant information. She was then able to work verbally, clear up the gynecological misunderstanding, and redeem her loss.

For other overeaters, diagnosis of a problem may come through patterns of movement. People may say that everything is fine, yet habitual gestures or postures reveal something else. The dance or movement therapist detects rhythmic patterns in small gestures or nervous habits, in breathing, pauses, reactions, and interactions. Tight muscle groups can be serving as emotional armor for an overeater, producing headaches, backaches, or cramps. The energy for these movements and unconscious bodily activities is connected to the unconscious mind, the defense mechanisms use psychic energy. An overeater can usually confirm the fact that the energy deriving from frustrated drives, instincts, and needs is used up in food orgies and binges. Such overeating may leave the body lethargic, lifeless, energyless—and also with no power to think about what is bothering the person.

Ellen, a young woman mentioned in some detail in Chapter 4, had a habitual gesture she made with her hands, spreading them out and down in front of her. It was the same gesture she used when she talked about spreading what she wanted to eat out on the table when she began her binges. The movement therapist asked Ellen if she felt like moving more of her body in the way her hands were moving. She did not feel any spontaneous impulse to move more. Ellen was, in fact, a soft-spoken person whose body usually remained relatively still. Instead of actually moving, she talked about what it would be like to move in the way her hands moved. She guessed it would be like diving down into a pool. The therapist placed pillows on the floor in front of Ellen and asked her to imitate that movement. Though nervous, she was eventually able to trust the experiment, slide forward and down onto the floor. Once there, she curled into a fetal position and said she was floating in the pool. All self-consciousness disappeared, and she began talking about how her parents had eagerly waited for her to be born, how they protected her and nurtured her. Ellen stayed curled up on the pillows as these relevant thoughts and memories flowed into consciousness at last.

The first business of dance or movement therapy is recognition on the therapist's part of movement patterns or themes that seem to be a real and recurrent part of the overeater's style or repertoire. The therapist then begins to work with the theme of that movement. This means exploring the movement, feeling it, living it more fully instead of denying it or making it stay imperceptible. Ellen's hand gestures had appeared often enough to elicit the therapist's attention. During therapy sessions Ellen herself eventually came to understand that her overeating was an attempt to submerge herself in a state of oblivion. She ate until she did not need to think, until she reached a stuffed stage of inactivity and could drift into sleep, without cares or responsibilities. She was trying to return to the peaceful "pool" she swam in before she was born into a world which had presented her with innumerable jobs and responsibilities to fulfill.

Rena, an overeater whose case appears in Chapter 5, began movement therapy by choosing the corner of a large soft couch to sit in when she came for sessions. But she sat almost immobile, her fists clenched. She tried to talk about her weight, but was inarticulate, and dug her fingernails into her palms. The therapist asked what else she might want to do with her fists, and she began pounding her thighs, and then the couch. The therapist asked her to go with the movement and see what else her hands wanted to do. Rena said she wanted to tear the room apart, including the stone fireplace. The therapist gave her a large stack of old telephone books and Rena sat on the floor in front of the fireplace and tore them into shreds. When she finished, she relaxed. Rena's face twinkled as she giggled about the "mess" she had made. During that session she had been given permission and encouragement to have her temper tantrum and make her mess. She was told not to clean up the shredded papers because such "messes" were perfectly permissible in the therapeutic setting.

The simple release of tension that came with the ripping activity served as an outlet for Rena. She felt relief and peacefulness when she was done, having dealt with her stress without resorting to the use of food. She reported back to us that for some time afterward her diet was very healthy and noncompulsive.

For Rena, mounting tension in her life aroused a need to dump her "load," or make a mess. But instead of letting go of these inner tensions that seemed dirty, messy, or destructive to her, she had been forcing herself to hold onto them. The food she compulsively pushed into her mouth had held the tensions down for so many years that she had become extremely obese. Finding a permissible way of letting go of the tension was therapeutic. But with nine children, five dogs, six cats, and a very strict and high-strung husband, it wasn't long before Rena found herself tense again. Much to her family's amazement, when such tense moments arose she would sit on the floor and rip up a large stack of old magazines: she had learned to find release and satisfaction in an activity that was both messy and safe on an occasion when she might otherwise have chewed a whole loaf of bread or a box of pastries.

Confronting a problem honestly yields beneficial results for the overeater. As people get to know their problems better, they can discover other modes of working with the problems, other resolutions for their tension. The experience of resolution is a clarification; with it comes amazement, peacefulness, and relief. For all the work involved in confronting the problem, there usually results an increase in energy. This new feeling of energy comes from the old energy that has been freed from the old defenses. The new energy increases self-esteem, and brings with it also an urge for continued growth—a form of self-love.

A young man, not previously mentioned in the book, was living his college years at home. Roger and his parents had determined that this was sensible economically, as their house was near enough to his college campus. But the young student soon found himself depressed, sleeping more and more, and eating more and more. He sought treatment with a therapist highly attuned to the use of movement and body language. The therapist began work by focusing on a small jerking movement Roger made with his right foot. He asked Roger to imagine what his foot really wanted to do. The jerking movement, which began as a small, nervous habit, gradually grew larger and evolved into a kick. This new movement became more and more violent, until it resembled a full-fledged temper tantrum. Roger was soon kicking and thrashing on the floor in an infantile behavior.

After emotionally experiencing several of these tantrums during sessions, Roger began in more verbal and intellectual ways to face the extent of his stored anger. He realized that he had very strong negative feelings about living at home—part of a lifelong pattern of passively accepting "reasonable" suggestions from his parents. Roger became more and more conscious of his repressed anger, delayed rebellion, and regression to oversleeping and overeating. His temper tantrums were reactions to his predicament, they resulted in a release of tension and renewed energy for his continued growth, including looking for his own housing. People who work through a feeling by going with it, exploring where it takes them, either verbally or in a movement pattern, report that they have a feeling of great relief afterward. Roger said he sometimes felt he was working his way through a fog, a maze, or a puzzle. His clear-headed feeling upon coming out of the fog was his excitement at seeing all the other possible ways to deal with the problems he faced.

Roger needed to discover for himself what the psychologically or emotionally powerful contingencies in his be-

168 · THE OVEREATERS

havior patterns were before attempting to control his overeating. When the powerful drive to overeat is part of an emotional need, external bribes or rewards are as futile as threats of punishment in effecting a cure. The energy involved in overeating needs to be expressed in new patterns or movements which will help the overeater discover what he is after, and how he can get it without having to binge. To really work, the rewards of *not* overeating must be personal and arrived at internally.

If overeating behavior is changed in such a way that fills a psychological need, the behavioral modification has a more lasting effectiveness. Of all the approaches to dieting, it has been found that behavior modification frequently has the best rate of success. Unfortunately, that success is usually not long-lasting unless a crucial psychological need has been met by the behavioral change. Effective behavior modification allows or suggests movement or activity which is closely connected to the overeater's emotional needs. In order to afford a real release and satisfaction, the activity must relate to the authentic core of the overeater's personality.

As we stated earlier, when movement therapy is used either diagnostically or as a form of behavior modification, the therapist's initial job is discerning the small, discrete movements that form the core pattern. For example, when Ellen (described in Chapter 4) began her treatment she had difficulty talking about her personal life. She was a long-term dieter and fortunately believed in exercises. During warm-up exercises in group sessions, she demonstrated which exercises made her feel good: Ellen liked the ones in which she could swing her arms in large arches, usually with her hands clenched in tight fists. Whenever she got to these exercises she expressed her pleasure. The therapist introduced more swings, showing Ellen how to add her shoulders, back, and torso to the motion.

Ellen soon built up a repertoire of exercises she could use that especially fitted her needs. For, in fact, this very ladylike person had never taken an aggressive stand with anyone. She had an indifferent husband, sons with school problems and one with a learning disability, a domineering mother-in-law, and her own sickly parents who doted on her. Ellen's delight in finding a safe way to swing her fists paralleled her need to lash out at these important and demanding people in her life—the core need probably being to unleash her childhood anger at two very dependent parents. When Ellen substituted a symbolic gesture which allowed her to fill some of her psychic needs, she discovered, on her own, a new way to handle some of her family tension. She was able to grab a coat after an argument at home and go for a walk, fast and furious, swinging her arms widely and with clenched fists. Ellen continued to diet, struggled with food binges, but her weight gain stopped. As she realized that she had some control over her compulsive eating, her self-esteem increased. By being able to express her emotions and feel better about herself, her anal tendencies dominated her less and less. She had turned her anger at her parents and her own family inward, only to find that she then hated her own bloated body. In this way, she never faced the original anger—not until she entered therapy did appropriate release occur.

A dance or movement therapist helps an overeater disentangle underlying feelings from others that are part of a socially acceptable emotional front. Ellen was alienated from the angry feelings in her body. She was unaware of her clenched fists, and needed tremendous encouragement to swing a punch, even when it was aimed at no one. When anger or sensuality or defiance are felt to be unpermissible, only small movements appear that hint at their existence—a clenched fist, a wink, a tapping foot. In a trusting therapeutic atmosphere a person can let out the small, hidden feelings. The movements get larger, clearer. He or she may be asked to try to evaluate what that part of the body is striving for through specific movement.[3]

Postures and Gestures: The Cases of Dolly and Nancy

Dolly, an overeater described in Chapter 3, was severely orally deprived. Her immaturity expressed itself in girlish gestures, attire, and habits of movement. She often rocked or swayed her body, or stroked her arm with her fingers. Her movements were slow and small, flowing and adapting to the environment, whether it was the chair or couch she curled up on or the wall behind her back. She liked foods she could suck, sip, lick, and consume slowly—sweet, soft foods that are packaged and sold for children or young people. She was continually reenacting behavior reminiscent of infancy, expressing herself primarily through these eating habits.

Dolly's treatment was one-to-one therapy with a movement specialist. She needed to experience a close relationship with a nurturing, supportive therapist and to establish the basic trust that first belongs to the mother-child relationship; she needed to regress to early stages of oral development. Only after Dolly was able to experience such closeness was she able to build some trust in herself.

The task of Dolly's therapy was to substitute her eating behavior with other behavior characteristic of the movements of the oral stage. Her treatment included some sessions in which Dolly and her therapist shared gestures, rocking rhythms, cradling postures, and gentle pumping movements in her arms. The rhythms were smooth and repetitive. Dolly preferred to do these "exercises" on the chair or the floor, where she felt safe, with less risk of falling.

She needed constant support, since she was not adventurous enough for impetuous movements and free-for-all exercises. Her movements had to feel safe and secure before she would go through with them. Behaviorally, she was reenacting her infancy. In time, she could verbally recall some of what her childhood had been like. The therapist encouraged her to pat or rub herself when she felt insecure, to move to "rock" music to build up her self-confidence, or even to ask her therapist for a massage when she wanted nurturing.

When she was given a chance to act out some of the rituals of birth and weaning, she emerged from her curled-up posture.[4] One of her exercises was to stretch her arms and legs while she was sitting, then to stand up and stretch her whole self. Such accomplishments were reflected in her day-to-day life by going out into the world and stretching a bit there, too. Significantly, she searched and found herself a job, which indicated the development of a more positive investment in herself. With this new kind of energy, Dolly was able to be more aggressive. She moved into her own apartment, away from her mother's house for the first time, even though she was already twenty-five.

She was trying to wean herself. But she needed tremendous amounts of support and encouragement, just as an infant does. When job, or income, or housing, or social connections did not *all* go well, Dolly retreated quickly to food and mother. Weight loss, as a consequence, was very slow. But even though the first few months of treatment did not show much loss of weight, they did show a significant increase in the kinds of behavior available to Dolly. As she experienced safety and security in therapy, she began to try new forms of more independent behavior.

At each stage of life, a child is learning a behavior pattern for meeting its needs. The energy for this behavior comes from a basic instinctual drive to grow. The first drive is directed toward survival and nourishment, and the first objects are food, the mother's breasts, and the nurturing figure itself. This is the oral drive, which is expressed in acts of grasping, pulling, rocking, sucking— all incorporative gestures moving from the environment inward toward the mouth. The second, anal drive is aggressively directed at objects that get in the way of having the child's needs satisfied and is evidenced by stomping, smashing gestures and by pushing outward toward the object standing in the way of its gratification. Every stage of development produces certain characteristic movements; it is the task of the movement therapist to use these typical patterns and rhythms as diagnostic tools.[5]

Nancy was a woman who spent years surrounding herself with layers of fat and cabinets of food. In treatment she was able to say that the only person who seemed to love her as a child had been her big fat grandmother. Nancy had not had enough of that love: her grandmother was not well, and her illness led to blindness and death. As Nancy remembered her, she also remembered her touch, because as the grandmother lost her sight she relied more and more on feeling Nancy's face and body to see how she was growing. She felt her fat loving arms and heard her grandmother's praises for the little rolls of fat on Nancy's own body—a sign that the little girl was getting plenty to eat. As Nancy talked about these memories she cried, longing for her loving grandmother. In the years since then Nancy had surrounded herself with her grandmother's soft, fat body.

In therapy Nancy often sat in a slumped position with her own big arms hugging herself just below her breasts. After several sessions that allowed Nancy to mourn the loss of love, she progressed to another stage of her own development: she began to get in touch with a different kind of memory. Nancy reconstructed all the ways in which her parents had kept her away from her grandmother. In her own family's house she never felt valuable or lovable and she used to beg to go live with Grandma. Her other relatives confused and frightened her. One man who was supposed to be an uncle had seduced her. When she told her parents, they were furious at her for letting it happen and made her promise to never tell. But at long last Nancy did begin to tell—in psychomotor therapy. In fact, she yelled and kicked and threw pillows and tried out all the vile, dirty language she could think of. The stiffled aggressive need to get even with the family that had deprived her of love and self-esteem exploded and retaliated. None of those people were actually present; she was safe in therapy to stomp on their fantasized faces. In one such session, Nancy was trembling from head to toe when she had finished her angry tirade.

During the weeks of treatment Nancy's appearance began to change. She began to carry herself differently. A new hair style, slimming clothes, some jewelry—these were manifestations of her new spirit of healthy survival. Her grandmother had finally died; but Nancy was alive, and vitality began to glimmer in her eyes and skin, and she developed a sparkle in her expression.

The socially acceptable forms of aggression, whether they are pillow fighting, yelling, or football games, are important, yet Nancy's family had denied her these needed outlets. People with no other way of being aggressive sometimes use eating for this purpose. Biting, for example, is a very primitive form of self-assertion. But eventually the destruction is directed against the self: biting, chewing, gobbling, gulping, and stuffing down food punishes the body with the discomfort and guilt of too much weight.

Overeaters who abuse their bodies in such ways are living as if they are not really one and the same as their own bodies. For them the real self is usually a younger or earlier version of who they think they are. The childhood needs are the important ones that they still harbor in their grown-up bodies. Sometimes it is the need to feel close to the feeding and caring person which can be seen in the need for sweets or the need to be fed frequently. The two-year-old's need to test independence, aggression, self-assertion, to try new accomplishments and get rewarded, can appear in later cravings to bite and chew and the use of food as a reward. The grown-up's actual physical body is therefore denied. Whether the body in fact needs the food is not considered, since the eating behavior is a response to emotional needs.

In dance or movement therapy the overeater is given a chance to identify with his long-denied physical self, become more aware of and accepting of its needs. The integrated personality finds a connection between the early childhood self and the adult self, its shape, form, and feelings. The road to integration can be frightening, painful, or sad, and people who are feeding the children in themselves sometimes ask "Won't my face get all wrinkled when I lose weight?" Acceptance of the life cycle—of time, growth, age, of gains and losses, dreams and reality—is a vital part of the process of integration.

DISCOVERING WHAT THE BODY NEEDS

The trouble with being trapped in an overweight body that one cannot identify with is that one does not really know what the body's needs are. The obese person lives in his head, where his other image of himself prevails. Lee, discussed in Chapter 5, lived with the needs of a little girl. She had been Mommy's helper, and that image predominated for several decades. Lee, who did not know the needs of her own woman's body, kept feeding the little girl inside herself. But all the while Lee was feeding that love-starved little girl, it was her adult body that kept getting more and more obese.

The theory of psychomotor therapy, which originated with Diane and Albert Pesso, suggests that the body's needs are best satisfied through interaction with others.[6] One may pat or stroke oneself, but the nervous tension behind this mannerism is not fully released until the individual finds interaction in a relationship that will fill the unspoken need to be touched. When Dolly (Chapter 3) felt separate or alone, she unconsciously stroked her forearm. The body has a need to be touched, stroked, petted, the senses in the skin crave stimulation. People with unconscious habits of twisting their hair or rubbing an arm or patting a thigh are sending out messages of unfulfilled needs that require action and interaction with others for their fulfillment. There are people who crave to be touched and held, who cannot permit themselves this pleasure; instead of reaching out for touch in an interaction with a person, a pet, or a gentle breeze on the skin, that desire is vehemently denied. They will permit food to come into their mouths, but the buried self cannot come out.

Other feelings need to get out, too. When angry feelings stay in, the tension inside the body causes the body pain. The adult body needs appropriate release of sexual tension. Even joy and excitement need expression: a shout, a skip, a twirl provide release that leaves the body free of tension. Joy, for example, cannot express itself when turned inward in the form of an ice cream cone; it turns instead to fat.

The body also has a need for rest. Yet it happens that many people do not always deal with that important physical need. They may try instead to get more fuel for themselves through food, overeating at the end of a difficult day and so giving the body the additional work of a difficult digestion. The food these people grab for energy is often heavy in carbohydrates; the sluggishness that follows allows them to rest without fear of an explosion of the tension buried under all that food. This is often the case with those people who are overcharged with nervous tension from their day's activities. The unreleased energy in their bodies is somehow fearful to them. They did not know how to release it properly during the day—perhaps it was anger or excitement as mentioned above—and they are afraid to relax in the evening because this tension may erupt.

When the mind is not in close touch with the body, the person lives inside ideas, thoughts, feelings, memories of feelings, worries, anxieties. His awarenesses are in his head, his body awareness minimized. Such a person does not like this body and does not really want to own it. He does not listen to his body's needs, being too overwhelmed by the needs of the self trapped inside. His movements appear to be either automatic or passive. Assertive, voluntary, willful movements are usually reduced and interactions avoided. The overeater alienated from his body does not skip when he is happy—he buys that ice cream cone instead. He does not fight when he is angry—he might pull at a piece of bread instead. Excitement and tension stay locked up inside and the need for self-expression is denied.

DEALING WITH THE BODY-IMAGE

The picture people carry around inside their heads about how they look and move is termed a body-image. People with weight problems usually develop body-image problems. Alienation—living inside the head and not the body—contributes to the distortion of body-image, as does dislike and rejection of the body, especially those parts that store fat. Body-image problems can be successfully treated with movement therapy because it is in action and interaction that the inner, feeling self and the outer, physical self can get to know one another and work together to fill mutual needs.

The image a person has of his body cannot always be corrected by a mirror, though that is a good place to begin getting information about the discrepancy between fantasy and reality. One woman carried in her head a picture of herself as obese. She used that distorted image to convey her feelings about herself, even though it was her mother who had been overweight. Yet even while she struggled to fight her minimal weight problem, she could not erase the mental image of herself as "fat." A man with all his extra weight stored in the middle of his trunk seemed unaware of his thin arms and legs. The mirror did not help, because as soon as he turned away from it, he returned to his "fat" feeling about himself, which he carried and concentrated in his midriff.

Distortion of body-image often involves boundary problems. "How big am I?" Overeaters who feel obese do not always know if they are five, fifteen, or fifty pounds overweight. Doubt and uncertainty haunts them; the bloated areas or parts that collect weight may seem so terribly powerful and overly important to the emotional existence of the overeater that fear of obesity is an obsessive concern. A woman wonders if her thighs look normal or enormous, a man wonders if his belly makes him look pregnant or tough. These confusions, their assessment and clarification, are a critical part of diagnosis and treatment of body-image problems.

When movement is experienced in the various parts of the body, it creates a vital feeling about that part. As body awareness is increased, new feedback and information can be integrated into the self-image: the awareness of the actions the muscles are taking, either their stretch or their contraction, is an important lesson in reality. Just as the mirror gives the real picture from the outside, the sense of movement gives the real picture from inside the body. The warmth, burn, pull, twist, of an action cannot be genuinely felt unless it is really happening.

For centuries, rhythm, chants, and dance rites have been used by mankind for their healing powers. Indeed, the movements made by the ancient medicine man are among the oldest forms of treatment. The common exaltation of the participants was felt in the release of tension, fear, and separateness.[7] Today movement and dance are being used by the medical profession to assist individuals in organizing and developing behavior which will enable them to satisfy their own internal needs as well as the demands of the external environment. For overeaters, the dualism of mind and body should always be explored and treated as an integrated unit.

10

---•---

Treatment

---•---

*A*n individual is a unique combination of the various psychological clusters we have thus far described. The first tool we use in the treatment of obesity is identifying the cluster complex of each overeater. Once diagnosis has been made it becomes more apparent what areas need attention in treatment.

ORAL CLUSTER

The oral cluster overeater is generally the most difficult to treat, since such a patient is likely to have the least developed sense of his or her own individuality. This type of overeater has strong needs to be closely linked or fused with a mother-figure. The predominant need for nurturance is acted out in overeating, an oral incorporation of maternal supplies. Because these supplies seem connected to survival itself, the hunger is often felt as desperation, which can lead to extreme obesity. This places the person in grave physical jeopardy. Though treatment requires a large investment of energy, it may literally be a life-saving investment.

Dealing with the eating behavior of the oral cluster overeater cannot by itself solve the overeating syndrome, since the focus on food supplies is tied directly to emotional issues. The core of such an overeater is emotionally starved. Treatment must deal with the intense need to fuse with mother, the nurturer. Confidence in the ability to survive independently must somehow be established, and a sense of self that can exist separate from the mother must be experienced. Treatment must offer an opportunity to develop this basic trust before eating behavior can really change. To illustrate how treatment can do this, we will look again at the case of Harry, the first presented in this book.

Harry was the most obese person we have ever treated. This treatment has been intermittent over the past six years. For the past two years, the course of treatment has been much more continuous and intense; Harry has steadily lost approximately 200 pounds. This has happened without hospitalization. Harry's amazing progress to date is the result of the energy invested in the relationship by his therapist.[1] This psychologist is a woman, which probably has facilitated his treatment to some extent, since the most severe deprivation of Harry's life was in the original relationship he had with his emotionally depriving mother.

Harry's therapist was able to become closely involved in his life, actively assuming the role of nurturing mother and feeding into the healthier parts of his personality. She visited him when he refused to leave his bedroom, wrote to him when he left town to try risking an actual trip, and arranged special weighing-in occasions on the particular type of scales needed to accommodate his enormous bulk. She managed to help with problems with his wife and children, and offered responsive feedback concerning his behavior and lifestyle. Harry came to trust his therapist as he had trusted no one else for the first thirty years of his life. Over the years he actually internalized some of her concern and involvement. He developed a new trust in himself and some sense of self-worth. This new outlook, which entailed trust in another and trust in himself, had to be built from scratch.

The psychologist gave Harry a life experience in which he had a new kind of care, something positive to replace the devastating negativism he experienced with his real mother. His basic hunger for security and nurturance was finally fed. In that way he was able to progress toward other stages of development. Instead of continually swimming in a sea of undifferentiated neediness, he began to form his own identity and self-esteem based on his more positive experiences. He learned to dare, to take a chance and come out of his womb-like bedroom, and to let go of some of the vast quantities of food he was hoarding there.

Harry needed to have treatment based on a central one-to-one relationship. Group therapy would have been inappropriate, since learning to deal with groups and to test one's identity in groups comes at later stages of development. With the oral cluster overeater, treatment must be geared to the earliest stage of development when the central issue in the life of a child is the nurturance from its mother.

The special kind of therapy from which Harry benefited is called one-to-one life involvement therapy—perhaps the single most effective treatment for oral cluster patients. Dolly, another oral cluster overeater, was also in one-to-one life involvement therapy. Because her original relationship with her mother had been extremely interdependent, mother and child had a fused identity. Her treatment was directed toward providing Dolly with opportunities to experience independence and develop a sense of her own personal identity. To do this, her therapist had to become involved in such questions as where

Dolly lived, what job opportunities she sought, and how she chose to spend her free time. As a caring, supportive, but undemanding figure, the therapist afforded Dolly an alliance in which she might grow.

At twenty-five, when Dolly began treatment, she was still living with her mother. Her therapist felt that Dolly would benefit from moving into an apartment of her own, and encouraged and supported this step, becoming actively involved in the details of moving while always showing respect and support for Dolly's own feelings and plans. When alone in her apartment Dolly was able to call her therapist, day or night, as part of her life involvement plan of treatment. She needed this new support system in order to exist separately from the original unhealthy system she had shared with her mother.

Although she worked for the first five months that she lived in her own apartment, Dolly had difficulty keeping her job—the first she had ever had in her life. When she lost that job, she became excessively frightened and overwhelmed by her feelings of inadequacy. Unemployment benefits were meager, and she panicked at the lack of real sources for supplies. She tried to look for a new job, but this additional stress was more than she was prepared to handle. At this point she chose her alliance with her mother over the alliance with her therapist that had been building. Dolly stopped therapy and abandoned her weight reduction program (under which she had lost a significant amount of weight). She went back home to mother after six months on her own.

In treating the oral cluster overeater, possible risks and benefits must be carefully weighed. The overeater and the professionals involved in the treatment must honestly answer several questions before proceeding: Is the weight problem severe enough (a genuine health hazard) to warrant stressful probing into the patient's psyche? Will this particular overeater be able to function in the face of such pressure? Is there a way to give this patient a sufficient amount of involved support while he or she diets? At times it is best to let the oral cluster overeater continue to use food for emotional support, even if it means remaining overweight. It may be that urging such a troubled person to find a new life and a new self may be asking too much.

ANAL CLUSTER

Treatment of an anal cluster overeater can be noisy, angry, tearful, frightening, and exciting. Overeaters who are using food to try to deal with issues that involve control, assertion, and shame have some very volatile exploration to do. Part of this exploration may be similar to going through the Terrible Two's again, struggling between holding on and letting go, vacillating between denial and assertion, dependency and independence. Treatment works best if it is structured to allow as wide an expression of these various and contradictory feelings as possible. Strong ambivalent feelings need to be unlocked, experienced, and analyzed; emotions that have been buried need to be brought to light and felt.

The expressive therapies (bioenergetics, psychodrama, primal therapy, etc.) are usually those that explore movement, dance, art, drama, music, play, and dreams. They augment the traditionally verbal process of psychoanalysis or psychotherapy eliciting a more unconscious level of participation. The anal cluster overeater can utilize these approaches quite profitably to get at buried material; with the release of pent-up emotion the anal patient experiences a gratifying lightening of the load of depression inherent in his condition.

Anal cluster overeaters tend to gulp down food—the objects of their aggressions get swallowed. Instead of having an effect on the world outside themselves, they affect their own bodies, stuffing themselves with unchewed and unassimilated food. The aggression is off-target and therefore unsatisfying. For that very reason it becomes compulsive.

Treatment, to be successful, must intervene in this cycle and provide a healthier outlet for the strong feelings.

Since the compulsive gulping results in alienating the outer body from the inner self, it is important to change this eating behavior. The alienation, symptomatic of the anal cluster overeater, is a poor defense mechanism for handling stress. Yet to change from gulping to chewing can be painful for the overeater: to chew slowly means to assimilate a part of the world, making it a part of the inner self. It is also a way of assuming responsibility for the action of overeating. By quietly chewing and assimilating the food, the overeater risks owning up to difficult emotions, such as aggression and anger.[2]

Our treatment of the anal cluster overeater always involves modifying gulping behavior. When disturbed feelings and a sense of pain come into the patient's awareness, instead of swallowing feelings, he is asked to experience them deliberately. It helps to write down or report the feelings that arise when the eater forces himself to chew instead of to gulp food. Feelings of disgust are common and need expression or discussion, since they are likely to be coming from the very heart of the anal patient's problem.

Let us look now at our treatment of Martin, described in Chapter 4. Martin was raised in a rigid home where his Christian Scientist parents denied his emotional and physical feelings. Martin was taught that his body was not truly real. Consequently, he developed a deep sense of alienation from his own anger and from his emotions in general. Martin gulped food down rapidly and overate, particularly during times of stress—those moments when he feared losing control and becoming irrationally angry. Overeating at those times was a form of control he imposed on himself to suppress his anger and avoid real action. He was trying to protect his inner self from acting on the anger. Whenever stress shook his self-esteem, he gulped down his food.

In treatment, Martin's propensity for compulsive behavior worked in his behalf. Since his diet allowed only 600 calories a day (he was warned that anything over 800 calories would increase his appetite), he was required to weigh his food carefully, even compulsively. He followed instructions to chew completely at least three mouthfuls of food at each meal and began to take responsibility for his actions and feelings. He found slow eating abhorrent and disgusting, probably because it unleashed a primitive sense of anger directed toward his parents.

His early world had given Martin an overdose of unwanted and unhappy experiences in the form of his parents' nurturance. By chewing food so carefully now he could no longer keep swallowing things the way they were: he had to deal with his anger and disgust at what he did not like.

This was a precarious period for Martin, for he was much closer to his feelings than ever before. If he met an undue amount of stress, it was not surprising that he had setbacks, and returned to his old overeating behavior. He needed supportive therapy while he dieted because he was getting closer to some very unhappy feelings.[3] His long-term tendency toward a sense of worthlessness and despair made him very vulnerable to failure.

The therapeutic use of antidepressants was begun. Martin's response was the most dramatic we have seen: he was able to diet until the drug was stopped, at which time he regressed to his earlier overeating behavior. Binging is a frequently sought solution to the anal patient's depressive tendencies. When the drug was restarted, he was at last able to diet and to deal with his emotional turmoil.

It is difficult to predict how well an anal cluster overeater will respond to antidepressants. If there is an indication of depression, and if the patient eats more when depressed, the use of antidepressants should be considered. Exercise also has an antidepressant effect and should be strongly encouraged in addition to, or even in place of, medication.

Martin needed supportive therapy that would allow him to express the feelings he was encountering. Due to his particularly self-conscious and withdrawn nature, he elected to do this on a one-to-one basis rather than in a group. The course of his treatment is interesting to follow because of the effect dieting and therapy had on the whole of his life: the ramifications surprised Martin and in the long run pleased him, even though the two years of his treatment were not easy for him.

At the beginning of treatment Martin claimed that his work as an engineer was the best part of his life. He felt the bosses at his corporation relied on him to solve their most difficult engineering problems. But he knew the corporation itself was not financially sound and that some workers were being layed off. After his dieting began, Martin was more in touch with his feelings of alienation, which changed his relationship with his corporation. At first he felt vulnerable and expendable; he worried that he too might be layed off. But his supportive therapy enabled him to maintain self-esteem. He gradually began to feel the company was using him. Martin became more expressive and more assertive. He felt he knew more about his business than his bosses. The corporation began to look less interesting to him and he started to search for a more responsible position.

At the same time, Martin began to date again. For the first time since his divorce, he considered the possibility that his broken marriage had not, after all, been his fault. A new blossoming of his sex life lead to genuine feelings of self-esteem. These new life experiences were, in a sense, a part of his ongoing expressive therapy. Manipulation of his diet enabled Martin to gradually return to and maintain an excellent, attractive weight. As he was giving up his protective layers of fat, he felt good. The new weight, which seemed more "desirable" to him, enabled him to expose himself more and more to women. His relationships as well as his self-esteem moved in a very positive direction.

For the past two years Martin has continued to do well. However, it must be realized that his early personality and defenses still exist. With stress, he could still regress. But the old, vulnerable self may be better able to remain in the background as time passes and as the new self acquires healthier ways of dealing with stress.

Treatment for Olga, another anal cluster overeater, involved antidepressant medication as well as a form of expressive therapy. Olga used the piano to indirectly express her anger at her alcoholic mother. She was eventually able to express this more directly, thereby learning more about herself. Olga was able to see that her dislike of herself, her feelings of low self-esteem and guilt, stemmed from her identification with her mother.

The particular form of expressive therapy that Olga underwent was psychomotor. This therapy, which worked well for her and others like her, originated with Albert and Diane Pesso.[4] She was helped to identify feelings she had about her "bad" mother and to construct an image of a "good" mother. Her sessions gave her opportunities to experience the loving and nurturing interaction she had always longed for.

The technique used to separate "good" and "bad" mother was quite simple and very effective. Working in a group, Olga structured a relationship that gave her a chance to feel and satisfy her memories, hopes, and fantasies about her mother. She was able to shout at her "bad" mother and feel effective when an accommodating figure cowered in response. Another "good" mother-figure stood by to give Olga whatever positive responses she asked for. She learned to ask her positive, accommodating "mother" to hold her hand, then embrace and hug her. In the embrace Olga's entire body relaxed as she lingered there, filling up on the positive interaction she had wanted so much.

Eventually Olga became aware of how much she had needed and wanted to scream and insult the drunken woman who had been her mother. She needed to kick and thrash at the negative mother as much as she needed to be held, rocked, praised, and patted by her positive mother. In psychomotor sessions Olga was able to physically go through these experiences—she felt the fears, hungers, and satisfactions in her body, in her muscles, in her breathing. Olga's self-assertion emerged with much pain and tender vulnerability to stress. As she got in touch with the pain, she needed protection. She spent over three years in further therapy, and only after the first full year was she able to actually take her coat off in sessions. Her therapist had to be always available to her, on a one-to-one level, giving support in times of crises.

For Olga, the crucial support was not verbal but through actions, through the actual experience of having support always there for her to turn to. In three years she lost 100 pounds. Her investment in therapy helped her maintain her struggling self-esteem, and she gradually internalized the nurturing relationship.

GENITAL CLUSTER

Chapter 5 describes overeating behavior when it is an expression of sexual desires and sexual identity. Overeaters in this cluster have a special task before they can diet successfully: they must attempt to explore and understand their feelings about sexuality with a sex counselor or other trained professional. Diet cannot be the only tool used by this type of overeater, since at best it will provide only temporary treatment for underlying problems in the genital character's development. A diet may even be part of the overeating binge: repentance after an orgy. The cycle of "sinning" by compulsive eating and repentance by compulsive dieting must be treated.

Many overeaters belonging to the genital cluster appear to be in a conflict about the perceived sexuality of their parents. The problem is most often reflected in a fusion of their own sexual identity with that of their mothers. Rena, Beth, Lee, Dave, and Morris all reflect this conflict.

We will begin with Beth's treatment. Her perception of her female sexuality was linked to having babies, since this was how she had perceived her own mother's womanhood. Beth, however, was unable to become pregnant. After many years of marriage, she underwent a thorough fertility work-up, at which point her sexual self-image—the infertile woman—caused her acute emotional anguish. This image conflicted with her mother's presentation of what womanhood stood for. Beth began to overeat compulsively, part of an attempt to fuse more successfully with her mother and to arrive at a closer connection with her childish perception of womanhood. By overeating she gained about thirty pounds, near the amount gained in a pregnancy. She was trying to affirm that she was a "real" female.

On a diet Beth did lose weight, but an interesting phenomenon occurred. She began to feel naughty, sexy, and sensuous. She felt feminine in a new and different way. Fantasies about men startled her; she had never had them before, and they seemed shameful to her. Beth's mother had never suggested ways of coping with any female role other than motherhood. By *not* becoming pregnant, by *not* overeating, Beth was dissociating herself from her mother's concept of womanhood. The diet was for her a dangerous experience that evoked uncertain feelings about her sexuality. Beth needed to incorporate her sexual desires into her concept of the family woman by heightening sexual gratification in her married life. By combining the two, she would come closer to being a whole, adult female.

Beth and her husband worked together with a sex therapist. The procedure was directive at the start. Each described their sex life in detail. Sexual fantasies were explored. The therapist made suggestions that helped to make intercourse more gratifying for the couple. Once a week husband and wife told the therapist how they felt about these new techniques and experiences. After only one month of therapy, Beth seemed more relaxed. Sexual fantasies about other men were less frequent and less disturbing to her. Her dieting took on a less compulsive aspect, and even without rigid adherence to it she was able to keep her weight fairly level.

Three years after this successful conclusion of therapy, Beth began feeling a recurrence of her overeating compulsion. Her weight started to go up again. Discussions revealed a new version of the old conflict in Beth's life: her husband was in the throes of making a decision to take a new job in a different city, and Beth felt the home she had created was in jeopardy. Her home had been an important part of her identity, but when it lost its feeling of security and permanence, the specter of her mother's concept of femininity—with all its domestic overtones—was again directly confronting her. She lost interest and pride in her house, threatened in her ability to create a good, stable home as evidence of her womanhood. Beth wanted to overeat again—her alternative way of reidentifying with her mother.

Up to this point, Beth had kept to herself her uneasiness about moving. The first step for her was to talk to her husband about how she viewed their possible move. Fortunately, when she did speak to him, he felt obliged to end his indecision: he gave the new job offer a final look, then decided to continue his present work in the same city. Beth's domestic life stabilized, interest and pride in her home returned quickly, and the urge to overeat subsided. As before, Beth needed to get in touch with her ambivalence about femininity, and how it affected her identity. She was then capable of dealing with family and home issues without substituting food for action.

Lee, also described in Chapter 5, underwent treatment

involving diet, exercise, and psychotherapy. She began by fasting for two weeks on a weight loss unit in a hospital. While there she began to use exercise and movement therapy techniques, and continued these as she adjusted to a 600-calorie diet. After she left the hospital, she maintained this diet for several weeks, but as her need for protein became more apparent (seen in some hair loss and brittle nails), the diet was raised to 800 calories. By keeping caloric count so low Lee's appetite diminished—a phenomenon noted in several nutritional studies. Lee stayed on the 600- to 800-calorie diet for six months, and lost a total of fifty pounds. For the past three years, she has maintained this weight loss and has also continued exercise and a psychotherapy program.

Lee's body-image was very negative. She was unhappy, and her fat was for her part of the ugliness that she used to explain her discontent. The strict dieting and initial weight loss made her feel happier. Even her breasts— emotionally charged parts of her body—were getting smaller. She enjoyed reducing the "ugliness" in herself: her mood was elevated, she felt new energy, a natural "high." Since it was important that she channel this physical energy, it was suggested she continue with her movement therapist. The form of exercise that worked best for her was a type of hatha yoga, which she used as part of her transition from compulsive eating to controlled dieting.

Lee's sensible exercising and dieting were newer, healthier ways of taking care of herself, and relied heavily on controls. In yoga she depended on almost daily sessions, moving in slow, sustained patterns with carefully regulated breathing. This control of the flow of breath and movement was part of her exploration of her own boundaries. She stayed away from impulsive movement, because she did not trust her impulses. (Overeating, it will be recalled, had been her primary defense against her frustrated sexual impulses.) Instead of losing awareness of the boundaries of her body by grossly extending them and bloating herself with food, Lee was now carefully redefining her boundaries. As her abdominal muscle tone improved through exercise, so too her outline of who she was in space became firmer. She organized her own yoga classes, which gave her another important form of control over her body, its activities and impulses.

Lee's psychotherapy afforded her an opportunity to explore the meanings of femininity. Food had been symbolic of maternal care, the nurturing breast, the form of womanhood with which she had identified. She had sought gratification of her own womanly needs in nurturance and feeding—she was the great giver. Feeding herself, as she fed others, had been her main outlet for self-gratification. Even to have sexual orgasm for her own pleasure was contrary to her ideal of a female identity. Dieting meant giving up these inappropriately emotional uses of food. This break with her old concept of nurturing femininity created a valuable opportunity for psychotherapy; it was the right time for exploring new meanings of femininity.

In psychotherapy Lee was encouraged to explore her female sexuality. She learned to masturbate herself, finding her own orgasm to be a source of pleasure that was not only enjoyable but available and permissible. She was encouraged to do things for her own sake, not always for others. She developed a feeling that she was worth something. Lee gradually left behind an old childhood burden: at one time her self-worth had seemed entirely dependent on her childish attempts to nurture and care for her little sister; now feelings of personal integrity at last became disengaged from that old role.

Dieting had given Lee a way to be adult, in control, independent of motherly feeding. Her yoga had helped her approach slimness and sensuousness without feeling out of control. In psychotherapy she got emotional support that affirmed for her the healthy quality of her new experience and that assured her that sexuality was a valid form of pleasure. At long last Lee was dealing successfully with the genital stage of development.

Morris, whose male identity was very deeply troubled,

also belongs to the genital cluster. All the phallic objects he surrounded himself with served to give him an aura of masculinity. He tried to compensate for his weaknesses with bravado, but underneath he had identified with his domineering mother. When Morris binged he was actually coming closest to acting out his inner feminine self: at such times he allowed himself to let go of his make-believe interest in women and lost interest in his symbols of male power. He stayed at home and became demanding, much as his own mother had ordered his father about all through Morris's childhood. When he binged, Morris ate phallic-shaped food with a passion, his mouth became a vagina and he a woman taking in a penis.

As we came to understand Morris's central psychodynamics, it became apparent that his sexual self-image was so distorted and bizarre that the possibility of a cure was in all likelihood out of the question. The fusion of his identity with that of his mother was unduly strong and pervasive. When distortion of sexual image is so extreme, as in Morris's case, it could be dangerous to try a cure that would leave the patient without abilities to cope. Extra weight is not necessarily life-threatening, and if overeating seems a crucial part of a person's coping mechanism, treatment can aim simply at preventing further weight gains and at furnishing supportive care.

Morris's health did endanger his life. He weighed 350 pounds and was only 5'7" tall. By the age of thirty-five he had had congestive heart failure twice, and his diabetes mellitus was becoming more difficult to control; his legs had become very swollen. He was admitted to the hospital in a hypersomolar coma with a blood sugar count of twelve hundred. Some form of treatment was imperative.

Morris was placed in a hospital obesity unit, and put on near total starvation for three weeks, given only large amounts of water and electrolytes. As Morris fasted, he began making passes at the nurses. His bravado, however, did not fool the hospital staff as he swaggered through the corridors with his fancy walking stick, giving out cigars and pens. Without being able to go on his effeminate binges, he returned to his super-male image.

As he was fasting, Morris was given the opportunity to establish a relationship with a male therapist. The therapist was highly experienced, but he found Morris difficult to treat with any conventional form of counseling. The therapist could not give support to Morris's real self because to do so would have provoked the binges which were a serious danger to Morris's health. The binges were in fact the moments when the less inhibited but terribly distorted self-image emerged. Morris had never met anyone who liked his demandingness or his binges, and he himself did not like this hidden self which erupted continuously. What came out at such times was the internalized mother who had consumed and bossed him.

A man who identifies so completely with his mother frequenty acts out this identity in homosexual relationships. But Morris could not stand to face his homosexuality, not only because of society's disapproval, but because of his own dislike for that part of himself. Therefore, the therapist had to support the bravado of Morris's male mask and his dieting. In the end, however, the distorted image had more power than the exterior controls and efforts: Morris's old binging behavior kept recurring, sometimes landing him back in the hospital for emergency care for diabetic shock. His weight loss program failed.

Reviewing Morris's tragic case, we wonder whether or not a different approach could have helped this man lose weight and lengthen the prospects of his staying alive. What if his therapist treated Morris like a son and became involved in his life? (We discussed the success of this form of one-to-one life involvement therapy at the beginning of the chapter.) Conceivably, Morris could have developed a new, healthier image of a father who is strong and yet warm. He may have been able to identify with the therapist and develop a sense of true self that he could like and not have to cover up. His own life experiences had never given him these opportunities. Could a therapist have saved him?

ADOLESCENT-ONSET CLUSTER

Treatment of the adolescent-onset overeater involves both social and sexual roles, the two primary areas of teenage development. In many cases the two are linked. The shape of the developing body is a prime concern of adolescents—feeling too tall or too short, feeling too voluptuous or not voluptuous enough, and so on. The teenager does not feel able to determine what is normal or natural for himself; he is in transition from holding up parental figures as authorities to becoming an adult with authority of his own. Rebellion and submission to authority are central issues which have not been resolved by young people who begin to overeat in adolescence; the overeating can represent either an excessive need to fuse or to separate from mother.

One of the most successful forms of treatment for overeaters who are still struggling with these adolescent concerns, no matter what their chronological age, is a particular form of behavior modification that allows them to relearn ways of feeding themselves. In the process they learn to know themselves, their impulses, appetites, and hungers in physical, social, and emotional ways. The skill developed in this program of behavior modification is primarily one of listening closely to cues from the body and responding to them. People are often taught to be sensitive to the needs of others and to satisfy them; young girls, in preparation for the roles of wives and mothers, are especially groomed to be sensitive in this way. Their social roles involve satisfying others' needs rather than their own. For a woman raised in this way, the skill of knowing her own needs is often left undeveloped. During treatment, such a woman gets to know herself better as she tries to tune into her appetite and to feed herself what she really wants to eat. She learns to know her real needs and to act on them, separating eating from her mother. Her career and social relationships are affected by her increased decisiveness on her own behalf and by her newly acquired sense of inner direction.

The major theme of this treatment is the self-definition involved in saying yes to foods that are important, and no to those that hold less attraction.[6] This form of self-definition is crucial to helping the adolescent overeater. Social pressures to eat, childhood voices about what to eat stored in the back of the memory, and guilt about cravings—all these interfere with self-determined choices. Overeaters in the adolescent stage of development are especially sensitive to social pressures. They are also in the middle of a struggle to separate from childhood controls and to move toward assertion of their own adult controls.

Most adolescent overeaters are very comfortable working in groups while they learn this new approach to food and hunger. Peer groups are especially beneficial to them: the members of the group are able to feel on an equal basis with one another, there is a healthy acceptance of responsibility for their own actions and choices. There is also a distinct move away from the family, as the self becomes the authority. For a doctor or dietician to prescribe a specific eating plan will certainly sabotage the important struggle to feed themselves. It is important to withhold any specific diet while the adolescent overeater gains skill in identifying the need to lick, chew, or suck. Is hunger felt in the belly, the throat, the mouth? How much is enough to satisfy the hunger for the time being? As sensitivity to these questions about the self are gained, a prescribed diet becomes less necessary for weight loss.

Bobbie, discussed in Chapter 6, was an adolescent-onset overeater. She was a thirty-seven-year-old teenager, full of strong rebellious feelings, narcissistic concern with her identity, sincere, intense, and very confused about her body. Even though she was only twenty-five to thirty pounds overweight, her body-image was of a person at least fifty pounds overweight. In her lifestyle she was continuously reenacting the adolescent problems that she had met more than twenty years before. Eating junk food was one of the ways she had of retaliating against her rigid, health-food-oriented mother.

Treatment for Bobbie was found in membership in a group aptly called Feeding Ourselves.[7] This group of women explored food awareness and body awareness issues in a ten-week series of meetings at which Emily Fox Kales, the founder of the group, functioned as a resource person. She offered tools of awareness, but each member of the group was her own authority on what was happening in her head and in her body. Each session involved an hour of physical movement and exercise, during which the members were encouraged not to use the mirror as an authority on how they were doing. Instead, they were asked to learn to trust their own bodies—how their muscles and joints were feeling rather than looking.

Bobbie began to blossom. She learned to stretch and turn, jump and leap without feeling awkward or self-conscious. Her movements became more emotionally expressive, and she was more able to articulate strong emotions in her body language. Instead of using junk food binges to deal with her feelings of unrest and rebellion, she acquired other tools for self-assertion.

Before grabbing food that beckoned to her from the candy stores, bakeries, and pizza shops she passed, or from her own refrigerator shelf, Bobbie began a new procedure: she tuned into what foods really "hummed" to her.[8] Did she find the idea of a candy bar appealing because of its chewy caramel? Or did she want the crunch of the nuts? Was it the sweet chocolate she wanted to lick? Being very specific about what foods were really important to her gave her a chance to assert her own choices in a very definitive fashion. She discovered that sometimes, for example, she wanted to chew on nuts, and didn't need the whole candy bar. She learned to assert this particular hunger, to turn her back on the beckoning candy bar, and to go find the nuts themselves. Her sense of entitlement was supported by her group: she could eat what really mattered to her without feeling guilty.

For Bobbie, eating habits changed without a prescribed diet. She ate what she felt she needed, often instead of regular meals. When her mother's forbidden junk foods were no longer forbidden, she lost the urge to cram them into herself all at one time; they were always there. She could eat greasy pizza instead of broiled chicken if she wished, and for a while she did just that. She was acting as her own authority, and she could make up her own mind.

None of these new skills were easy for Bobbie to acquire. Trial and error meant there were still some binges, still some overeating, and still more guilt, frustration, and confusion to experience. Though eventually she lost some weight, she followed no miraculous reducing diet. In the group she was in, no one weighed her, no one counted her caloric intake or defined her diet. Instead, group members offered strength and support. They were other women whose image she could identify with, women similar to her. At times these women offered her advice, opinions, even some mothering. But there was no ultimate authority figure in the group. Her archaic image of an authoritarian mother lost its power over her. In the months that followed these group sessions, Bobbie continued to experiment with self-regulation. Eventually, she did not need junk foods as a symbol for her independence; without binging, her weight dropped easily.

ADULT-ONSET CLUSTER

The adult-onset overeater also requires a particular approach in treatment. When an adult finds that overeating has become a part of life, not just a temporary or occasional event, the first question to consider is "What changed?" What has happened in the person's life, what is different in the demands of his environment? The overeater must begin his treatment program by looking for a significant interruption or change in lifestyle or cimcumstance. The overeating is likely to be his way of adapting to these new circumstances, yet it is maladaptive behavior, since instead of finding a solution to the problem that has arisen in his lifestyle or environment, he is creating a weight problem for himself as well. Identifying the change in his circumstances may lead to a more adaptive way of handling the underlying problem.

Sometimes large amounts of food are simply part of an old eating pattern, and the only discernible change in circumstance is a decrease in physical activity as the person ages. The result is a weight increase. The eating behavior, once adaptive, is now maladaptive. If physical activity cannot return to its previous level, as frequently happens when a more sedentary lifestyle is connected to aging, then the maladaptive eating has to change. This change may not seem dramatic: for example, something as small as having a dozen french fries at lunch each day can add up to eighteen pounds of fat in a year. Omitting the french fries is sensible behavior modification. So is burning up the extra 200 calories they have by adding a two-mile walk to the person's after-lunch routine.

Treatment of adult-onset overeating is often connected to other types of changes, not merely habitual intake of extra calories or the reduction of exercise. Sometimes changes in needs and circumstances are related to emotional tensions, as when an adult stress arises, and the person has difficulty dealing with it in an appropriately mature fashion. The adult may partly regress to the oral, anal, genital, or adolescent stage instead of dealing with the adult stress and tension. Successful treatment requires finding an adequate solution to the present problem so that the overeater can give up the inadequate and archaic solution of overeating.

When Millie, the adult-onset overeater described in Chapter 7, lost her closeness to her husband because he put a stop to their sex life, she did not deal with the problem in a mature way. Instead of seeking gynecological assistance or sexual counseling for the two of them, she began to console herself for her loss by overeating. This solution, of course, did not help her sex life at all. Correction of Millie's weight problem meant careful diagnosis of what had changed in her life at the time her overeating appeared. Millie and her husband received counseling from her doctor and learned that sexual intercourse would not cause her previous cancer of the cervix to recur. Knowledge of this fact allowed her sex life and intimacy with her husband to resume. Millie lost weight without even trying.

One woman found that each time she was preparing food for her husband or one of their four children, she also fed herself. Three meals a day for the six people in her family amounted to eighteen meals, as many as eighteen possible nibbles for her. To solve the problem behaviorally, she was asked first to record what she ate, when, where, and in what mood. By keeping track of exactly what she put into her mouth and what her mood was at that point in the day, she learned that when she was annoyed or frustrated by either her husband or her children, she took very generous nibbles for herself. The more tension there was in the house, the bigger were her treats for herself. If the children were noisy or unruly, she would eat one of the sandwiches she had been making for them. This did not quiet the children, nor even teach them to control their boisterous activity. Speaking to the children and giving vent to her anger would have been a more on-target use of her mouth than eating had been.

Note taking—of time, place, mood, and specific food—can be a valuable tool for understanding how overeating is functioning in the lifestyle of a person, since it brings about awareness of the use of eating behavior—the first step in modifying it. Other techniques of behavior modification are also helpful.[9,10] A salesman found that at business lunches he was eating quickly and compulsively as the tensions of making transactions mounted. He was advised to modify his eating behavior by putting his fork down between each bite. A housewife found that the meals she had during an otherwise routine day were one of her main sources of entertainment and interest. She was advised to use smaller plates for smaller portions, and to repeat the same foods over and over again, adding variety only by alternating the spot where she would sit and the place setting she chose for herself.

In general, these rather mild techniques of behavior modification are more useful and successful for the person whose overeating is not closely grounded to an emotional conflict. For Millie, whose overeating was connected to loss of fusion with her husband, new factual information made it possible for her to modify her eating behavior. But in most cases where overeating is related to emotional conflict, one has to do more than simply provide new information. However, even in these more difficult cases techniques of behavior modification can provide some solace to the overeater, sometimes allowing for weight loss while the more difficult issues are being tackled. Furthermore, the weight loss can be helpful in exposing the patient to the areas of his vulnerability, eventually making him more amenable to needed psychotherapy.

When an adult's life changes by becoming more isolated or lonely, overeating can become a way of trying to fill the emptiness. Losing a loved one, having children or family or friends move away, or entering a strange neighborhood —all these can induce loneliness, boredom, and self-pity.

Overeating may appear in an attempt to deal with the problem of fusion or lack of closeness. In cases like this, counting calories is not the solution to the problem. Increasing social contacts is more relevant to self-esteem and helps to fill the hunger for self-worth and involvement. Overeating is essentially a solitary act; an activity that involves an interaction between people, such as quieting the children when they are noisy, or seeking sexual counseling with a partner, is more likely to solve problems. Therapist, doctor, or counselor can serve as a type of social director, encouraging modification of behavior so that social factors in the patient's life improve. This can be a central aspect of behavior modification.

SOCIAL FACTORS

Social factors are an important, even crucial, consideration in the treatment of overeating. Since the most influential social elements are the earliest ones, approaching the eating problems of childhood by influencing the early social situation promises to be an effective form of preventive treatment. The mother and father, the immediate family, the extended family, and the subculture are strong determinants of the quality of the eating experience. When social factors can be spotted as contributing to overeating, the social experiences can be manipulated in an attempt to eradicate this behavior.

Mothering that is excessively involved in feeding, frequently a part of the Momism syndrome, can lead to overeating. Family interactions centered on food sharing and meal times reinforces the concept of fusion through food. Too, prophetic projections of images onto children tend to be self-fulfilling: using favorite foods and eating patterns as a way of characterizing and individualizing children restricts them for life.

Finally, infants and children need to be prepared for living in a Demand Culture. Since food is readily accessible, upon immediate demand, and since people are able to act out their hungers and replenish their needs with fewer obstacles than ever before, a new sensitivity to food is required. Knowing what one's hungers and needs really are and responding to internal instead of external clues are imperative for sanely balanced eating in a culture that offers immoderate amounts of consumerism—often in the form of food.

Michelle's case was discussed in Chapter 8, dealing with social factors in the problem of obesity. Her family had given her only one important and prophetic message—to eat well and stay healthy, safe, and pretty. Being pretty meant smiling sweetly. Being safe meant sitting or walking, never running or jumping or risking physical exertion. Being healthy was especially central because her mother was chronically ill. By overeating Michelle showed her parents that she was well; no other ways of coping with stress were suggested to her.

Michelle's treatment involved several stages of growth after she left home. She was partially able to overcome her early socializing experiences through assertiveness training, consciousness raising, group support, beauty counseling, and exercise techniques. Her ways of coping expanded as she focused on these different areas. She was able to modify her behavior, to find new ways to deal with stress, and to curb her overeating. Nevertheless, though the techniques were effective, they were external, and never fully incorporated into Michelle's identity.

To affect the socialization process in positive ways means intervening in the critical milestones of development. The adult overeater carries within him the history of oral, anal, genital, and adolescent stages of development, and where the roots of his eating problem rest determine what form of treatment is indicated. By understanding the cluster of each patient one can proceed to treat each patient as an individual, instead of lumping all fat people and overeaters together.

Notes

CHAPTER 2

1. Rose, G. A., and Williams, R. T.: "Metabolic studies on large and small eaters." *Br. J. Nutrition,* 15:1, 1961.

2. Bray, G. A.: "Effect of diet and trilodothyronine on the activity of sn-glycerol-3-phosphate dehydrogenase and on the metabolism of glucose and pyruvate by adipose tissue of obese patients." *J. Clin. Invest.,* 48:1413, 1969.

3. Ismail-Beigi, F., and Edelman, I. S.: "Mechanism of thyroid calorigenesis: Role of active sodium transport." *Proc. Nat. Acad. Sci.,* 67:1071, 1970.

4. Quaade, F.: "Insulation as a creative and maintaining factor in leanness and obesity." *Energy Balance in Man* (M. Apfelbaum, ed.), Paris, Masson et Cie., 1973, pp. 135–140.

5. Young, J. B., and Landsberg, L.: "Stimulation of the sympathetic nervous system during sucrose feeding." *Nature,* 269:615, 1977.

6. Miller, D. S., and Mumford, P.: *Energy Balance in Man* (M. Apfelbaum, ed.), Paris, Masson et Cie., 1973, pp. 195–207.

7. Sims, E. H., Danforth, E. H., Jr., Horton, E. S., Bray, G. A., Glennon, J. A., and Salans, L. B.: "Endocrine and metabolic effects of experimental obesity in man." *Recent Prog. Horm. Res.,* 29:457, 1973.

8. Bray, G. A., Raben, M. S., Londono, J., and Gallagher, T. F., Jr.: "Effects of triiodothyronine, growth hormone, and anabolic steroids on nitrogen excretion and oxygen consumption of obese patients." *J. Clin. Endocrinol.,* 33:293, 1971.

9. Ball, M. F., El-Khodary, A., and Canary, J.: "Growth hormone response in the thinned obese." *J. Clin. Endocrinol. Metab.,* 34:498, 1972.

10. Balagura, S.: "Neurophysiologic aspects: Hypothalamic factors in the control of eating behavior." *Advances in Psychosom. Med.,* 7:25, 1972.

11. Leibowitz, S. F.: "Brain catecholaminergic mechanisms for control of hunger." *Hunger: Basic Mechanisms and Clinical Implications* (Novin, D., Wyrwicka, W., and Bray, G. A., eds.), New York, Raven Press, 1975.

12. Mayer, J.: "Glucostatic mechanism of regulation of food intake." *New England J. Med.,* 249:13, 1953.

13. Debons, A. F., Silver, L., Cronkite, E. P., Johnson, H. A., Brecher, G., Tenzer, D., and Schwartz, I. L.: "Localization of gold in mouse brain in relation to gold thioglucose." *Am. J. Physiol.,* 202:743, 1962.

14. Hirsch, J., and Han, P. W.: "Cellularity of rat adipose tissue: Effects of growth, starvation and obesity." *J. Lipid Res.,* 10:77, 1969.

15. Brook, C. G. D., Lloyd, J. K., and Wolf, O. H.: "Relationship between age of onset of obesity and size and number of adipose cells." *Br. Med. J.,* 2:25, 1972.

16. Faust, I. M., Johnson, P. R., Hirsch, J.: "Noncompensation of adipose mass in partially lipectomized mice and rats." *Am. J. Physiol.,* 231(2):539, 1976.

17. Mellinkoff, S. M., Frankland, M., Boyle, D., and Greipel, M.: "Relationship between serum amino acid concentration and fluctuations in appetite." *J. Appl. Physiol.,* 8:535, 1956.

18. Wise, J. K., Hendler, R., and Felig, P.: "Evaluation of alpha-cell function by infusion of alanine in normal, diabetic, and obese subjects." *New England J. Med.,* 288:484, 1973.

19. Campbell, R. G., Hashim, S. A., and Van Itallie, T. B.: "Studies of food-intake regulation in man: Responses to variations in nutritive density in lean and obese subjects." *New England J. Med.,* 285:1402, 1971.

20. Schachter, S.: "Obesity and eating. Internal and external cues differentially effect the eating behavior of obese and normal subjects." *Science,* 161:751, 1968.

21. Schachter, S., and Gross, L. P.: "Manipulated time and eating behavior." *J. Personality Soc. Psychol.,* 10:98, 1968.

CHAPTER 3

1. Erikson, E. H.: "Identity and the life cycle." *Psychological Issues,* monograph, 1959.

2. Erikson, E. H.: Eight Ages of Man. *Childhood and Society,* 2nd ed., New York, W. W. Norton and Co., 1963, pp. 247–269.

3. Bruch, H.: "Hunger and instinct." *J. Nerv. and Ment. Dis.,* 149:91, 1969.

4. Fenichel, O.: Development of Instincts, Infantile Sexuality. *The Psychoanalytic Theory of Neurosis,* New York, W. W. Norton and Co., 1972, pp. 62–66.

CHAPTER 4

1. Fenichel, O.: *The Psychoanalytic Theory of Neurosis,* New York, W. W. Norton and Co., 1972, pp. 66–68, 176, 278–310.

2. Perls, F., Hefferline, R. F., and Goodman, P.: *Gestalt Therapy,* New York, Dell Publishing Co., 1951, pp. 199–208.

3. Erikson, E. H.: The Theory of Infantile Sexuality. *Childhood and Society,* 2nd ed., New York, W. W. Norton and Co., 1963, pp. 48–108.

CHAPTER 5

1. Fenichel, O.: Organ Neuroses. *The Psychoanalytic Theory of Neurosis,* New York, W. W. Norton and Co., 1972, pp. 240–242.

2. Fenichel, O.: Development of Instincts, Infantile Sexuality. *The Psychoanalytic Theory of Neurosis,* New York, W. W. Norton and Co., 1972, pp. 74–83.

3. Erikson, E. H.: The Theory of Infantile Sexuality. *Childhood and Society,* 2nd ed., New York, W. W. Norton and Co., 1963, pp. 85–108.

CHAPTER 6

1. Erikson, E. H.: Youth and the Evolution of Identity. *Childhood and Society,* 2nd ed., New York, W. W. Norton and Co., 1963, pp. 275–393.

2. Mayer, Jean: Obesity in Adolescence. *Overweight Causes, Cost, and Control,* Englewood Cliffs, Prentice-Hall, 1968, pp. 116–130.

3. Freud, A.: *The Ego and the Mechanisms of Defense,* London, Hogarth Press, 1937.

4. Mayer, J.: p. 117.

5. Bruch, H.: "Eating disorders in adolescence." *Proc. Am. Psychopath. Assoc.,* 59:181, 1970.

6. Bruch, H.: "Obesity in childhood and personality development." *Am. J. Orthops.,* 11, 1941.

CHAPTER 7

1. Lowe, C. R., and Gibson, J. R.: "Changes in body weight associated with age and marital status." *Br. Med. J.,* 2:1006, 1955.

2. Bray, G. A.: Experimental and Clinical Forms of Obesity.

The Obese Patient, Philadelphia, W. B. Saunders Co., 1976, pp. 203–205.

3. Erikson, E. H.: Eight Ages of Man. *Childhood and Society,* 2nd ed., New York, W. W. Norton and Co., 1963, pp. 266–268.

CHAPTER 8

1. Ravelli, G. P., Stein, Z. A., and Susse, M. W.: "Obesity in young men after famine exposure in utero and early infancy." *New England J. Med.,* 295:349, 1976.

2. Erikson, E. H.: *Childhood and Society,* 2nd ed., New York, W. W. Norton and Co., 1963.

3. Joffe, N. F.: "Food habits of selected subcultures in the United States." *Bull. Nat. Res. Council,* 108:97, 1943.

4. Goldblatt, P. B., Moore, M. E., and Stunkard, A. J.: "Social factors in obesity." *JAMA,* 192:97, 1965.

5. Keys, A.: "Coronary heart disease in seven countries." *Am. Heart Assn. Monograph #29,* April, 1970.

6. Lee, D.: Cultural Factors in Dietary Choice. *Freedom and Culture,* Englewood Cliffs, Prentice Hall, 1959, pp. 154–161.

7. Erikson, E. H.: Reflections on the American Identity. *Childhood and Society,* 2nd ed., New York, W. W. Norton and Co., 1963, pp. 288–298.

8. Boskind-Lodahl, M. "Cinderella's step-sisters: A feminist perspective on Anorexia Nervosa and Bulimia." *Signs: J. Women in Cult. and Soc.,* 2:342, 1976.

9. Marcus, Mary G.: "The Power of a Name." *Psychology Today,* Vol. 10, No. 5, pp. 75–78, October, 1976.

10. Fifty-nine percent of children were obese before the age of three in families where there was obesity in more than one relative in the immediate family. Only thirty-one percent of children were obese before the age of three in families where none or at most one relative was obese. *See* Mossbery, H. O.: "Obesity in children: A clinical-prognostical investigation." *Acta Ped.,* 35:Suppl. 2, 1, 1948.

11. Stunkard, A. J., d'Aquili, E., Sonja, F., and Fillon, R. D. L.: "Influence of social class on obesity and thinness in children." *JAMA,* 221:579, 1972.

12. Mayer, J.: Social Attitudes and the Obese. *Overweight Causes, Cost, and Control,* Englewood Cliffs, Prentice-Hall, 1968, pp. 84–91.

CHAPTER 9

1. Lowen, A.: *The Betrayal of the Body,* New York, Collier Book Co., 1969, pp. 145–160.

2. Perls, F., Hefferline, R. F., and Goodman, P.: *Gestalt Therapy,* New York, Dell Publishing Co., 1951, p. 288.

3. Pesso, A.: *Movement in Psychotherapy: Psychomotor Techniques and Training,* New York University Press, 1969.

4. Bernstein, P. L.: *Theory and Methods in Dance-Movement Therapy,* Dubuque, Iowa, Kendall Hunt Publishing Co., 1975, pp. 190–112.

5. *Ibid.,* p. 90.

6. Pesso, A.: *Experience in Action: A Psychomotor Psychology,* New York University Press, 1973.

7. Bernstein, p. 3.

CHAPTER 10

1. Shapiro, Faye, Ph.D., Life Involvement Institute, Cambridge, Mass.

2. Perls, F., Hefferline, R. F., and Goodman, P.: Introjection. *Gestalt Therapy,* New York, Dell Publishing Co., 1951, pp. 189–210.

3. Stunkard, A. J., and Rush, J.: "Dieting and depression reexamined." *Annals Internal Med.,* 81:526, 1974.

4. Pesso, A.: *Experience in Action: A Psychomotor Psychology,* New York University Press, 1973.

5. Stunkard and Rush, p. 530.

6. Pearson, L., and Pearson, L. R.: *The Psychologist's Eat Anything Diet,* New York, Popular Library, 1976.

7. Feeding Ourselves, 6 Bartlet Street, Arlington, Mass. 02174.

8. Pearson and Pearson, pp. 13–14.

9. Harmatz, M. G., and Lapuc, P.: "Behavior modifications of overeating in a psychiatric population." *J. Consult. Clin. Psych.,* 32:583, 1968.

10. Penick, S. B., Fillon, R., and Fox, S.: "Behavior modification in the treatment of obesity." *Psychosom. Med.,* 33:49, 1971.

Index

Adolescent-onset overeater
cluster, 106–115
case histories, 109–112
dynamics of, 106–109,
112–115
treatment for, 194–197
Adrenal gland, overactive,
24–25
Adult-onset overeater cluster,
116–133
case histories, 117–123,
125–132
diagnosis of, 120–121
dynamics of, 116–117,
123–125, 132–133
housewives in, 123–127
treatment of, 198–201
Advertising, overeating and,
137–138
Aggression, anal cluster and,
182–184
See also Anger
Alcoholism, parental, 62–63,
80–84, 88
Amphetamines, 28, 37

Anal cluster overeaters, 58–85
adult-onset overeating and,
118–119
case histories, 69–84
dance-movement therapy
and, 171–172
dynamics of, 58–69, 84–85
treatment for, 182–187
Anger
dance-movement therapy
and, 161–162
overeating and, 118
suppression of, physical
problems caused by,
175
Anorexia nervosa
Momism and, 145–146
physiologic causes, 114–115
Antidepressants, 68–69, 184
Appetite
amphetamines and, 28
steroid stimulation of, 25
See also Appetite regulation
Appetite regulation, 34–43
antidepressants and, 68–69

body fat cells and, 39–40
demand feeding and, 156
homeostasis and, 38–39
neurotransmitters and,
    34–36
ATP production, basal
    metabolism and, 21–23, 24

Basal metabolism, 21–23
of obese and nonobese
    patients, 21
thyroid hormone and, 23–24
See also Metabolism
Behavior modification
in adolescent-onset cluster,
    194–197
movement therapy as form
    of, 168
obesity and, 42–43
Binges, 129
by anal cluster patients,
    65–66, 76–77
by children, 16–17
Blood sugar levels, 25–26, 38
Body-image, 92–93, 129
in adolescence, 108–109
of anal cluster patients,
    61–62, 70
dance-movement therapy
    and, 190
overeating and, 173–174,
    176–177
Body needs, 174–176

Caloric intake, appetite
    control and, 17–19, 41
Career women, overeating by,
    128–132
Case histories
of adolescent-onset
    overeaters, 109–112
of adult-onset overeaters,
    117–123, 125–132
of anal cluster overeaters,
    69–84

of dance-movement
    therapy, 161–174
of oral cluster overeaters,
    47–57
of self-fulfilling prophecy,
    148–150
Catecholamines, 28–32, 35–37
Childhood development
anal stage of, see Anal
    cluster overeaters
body movement and, 158
classification of overeaters
    by stages of, 13–14
oral stage of, see Oral
    cluster overeaters
Children
eating behavior of, 131, 135,
    152–154
hypothyroid, 23–24
obese, fat cells of, 39–40
subcultural attitudes
    toward obesity in,
    140–141
See also Childhood
    development;
    Mother-child relations;
    Parent-child relations
Cold stress, metabolic
    response to, 29–30
Compulsive activity, 159–160
Compulsive eating, 187
Cortisone, weight gain and,
    24
Crash diets, 129
Cues, external and internal,
    41–42

Dance-movement therapy,
    157–177, 190
body-image and, 176–177
case histories of, 161–174
diagnosis of overeating
    problem with, 171–172
discovery of body needs
    with, 174–176

theory of, 11, 12, 157–161
Definitions of obesity, 19
Demand feeding, overeating
    and, 139–140, 156, 201–202
Diabetes, 26, 38
Diet-induced thermogenesis,
    weight gain and, 30–32
Dieting (Diets)
    and adolescent-onset
        overeaters, 111–112, 195
    and anal cluster patients,
        65, 66–67
    blood sugar and, 26
    classification of overeaters
        and, 13–14
    and genital cluster
        overeaters, 187
    and weight loss of obese
        and nonobese patients,
        20–21
    See also Low-carbohydrate
        diet
Disgust, development of,
    60–61

Eating behavior
    changes needed in, 155–156
    cyclical patterns of, 16–17
    intervention in, 196–197,
        201–202
    parental attitudes and,
        148–150
    society and, 134–140
Emotional closeness,
    overeating and, 137–138,
    141–142
Emotional problems
    classification of overeaters
        by, 12–14
    overeating and, 42–43
    physical movement and,
        158, 161
    treatment of adult-onset
        overeating and, 198–199

Exercise
    and depression in anal
        cluster overeaters, 184
    diet-induced thermogenesis
        and, 31
    See also Dance-movement
        therapy; Physical
        movement
Expressive therapies, 182–187
External cues, 41–42, 138–139

Famine. *See* Food deprivation
Fasting, and blood sugar
    levels, 26
Fat cell hypothesis, 39–40
    and fetal food deprivation,
        135–136
Feeding behavior. *See* Eating
    behavior
"Feeding Ourselves," 196–197
Fluid loss, 20–21
Food
    emotional closeness and,
        137–138, 141–142
    style of serving, 128,
        130–131
    See also Eating behavior
Food binges. *See* Binges
Food deprivation, 135–137
Food intake
    fluctuations in, 16–17
    and food storage, 21–22
    hypothalamic
        catecholamines and,
        36–37
    metabolic response to cold
        stress and, 30
    note-taking on, 199–200
    See also Binges; Eating
        behavior; Overeating
Force feeding, weight-gain
    studies and, 31–33

Generativity, 127
Genital cluster overeaters,
    86–105

case histories, 88–104
dynamics of, 86–88, 104–105
treatment for, 187–194
Glandular disorders. *See*
Adrenal gland;
Hypothyroidism;
Stein-Leventhal syndrome
Glucagon, blood sugar and, 38
Glucostat, 39
Glycogen storage, 21–22, 23
Group therapy, 11–112, 115,
178–182
Growth hormone, 33–34
Gulping behavior, 61, 76,
126–127, 182–183

Heredity, localized obesity
and, 19–20
Hoarding behavior, 49
Homosexuality, latent,
193–194
Hormones. *See*
Catecholamines; Growth
hormone; etc.
Housewives, 123–125, 199–200
Hunger center of
hypothalamus, 34–35
Hypothalamus, 34–35, 36
Hypothyroidism, 23–24, 28

Identity conflicts
marriage and, 123–124
overeating and, 106,
129–130
Infant feeding, 137, 139–140,
152–154
Infantile behavior, 167,
170–171
Insulin, 25–26, 38
Internal cues, 41

Lipostat, 39, 40, 41
Localized obesity, 19–20
Low-carbohydrate diet, 20–21

Menstruation,
Stein-Leventhal syndrome
and, 25
Metabolic disorders, "new,"
27–34
Metabolism
cold exposure and, 29–30
growth hormone and, 32–34
overeating and, 16
pheochromocytoma and,
27–28
See also Basal metabolism
Metropolitan Life Insurance
Company tables, 19, 29
Momism, 201
anorexia nervosa and,
145–146
overeating and, 142–146
Mother-child relations
in adolescence, 109–110
anorexia nervosa and,
114–115
oral cluster and, 45–47,
54–56
See also Momism;
Parent-child relations
Motherhood, weight problems
and, 124–125, 129
Movements and overweight,
18

Neurotransmitters, appetite
control by hypothalamus
and, 34–36
Nurturing, overeating and,
148–152, 178–182

Obesity. *See* Overeating
One-to-one involvement
therapy, 178–182
Oral cluster overeaters, 44–57
case histories, 47–57

and dance-movement
therapy, 170–172
dangers of treating, 181–182
dynamics of,45–47, 51–52,
113–114
and food deprivation, 135
treatment of, 178–182
Overeating
advertising and, 137–138
appetite control and, 41–42
children and, 16–17, 137
classification of, 12–13
dance-movement therapy
for, *see* Dance-
movement therapy
deficient hypothalamic
catecholamine release
and, 35–36
defined, 19
diabetes and, 26
diseases leading to, 20–27
distorted body-image and,
176–177
emotional problems and,
42–43
food deprivation and,
135–136
as habit, 116–117
low blood sugar and, 25–26
medical causes of, 15–43
Momism and, 142–146
"normal," 16–17
self-image and, 151
society and, *see* Society
stress and, 16, 116
and sympathetic nervous
system, 32
treatment of, *see* Treatment
of overeaters
weight gain and, 17–19
See also Adolescent-onset
overeater cluster;
Adult-onset overeater
cluster; Anal cluster

overeaters; Genital
cluster overeaters; Oral
cluster overeaters

Parent-child relations
in adolescence, 106–108
and adult-onset overeating,
121, 128, 129
and anal cluster overeaters,
69–70, 71, 74–75, 76
and self-fulfilling
prophecies, 146–152
See also Mother-child
relations
Phenochromocytoma, obesity
and, 27–28
Physical activity
caloric requirements and,
18–19
decrease in, 117, 119–120,
198
emotional meaning of,
157–161
See also Dance-movement
therapy
Pregnancy, food deprivation
during, 135–137

Satiety centers of
hypothalamus, 34–35
Schedule feeding, 152–154
Self-fulfilling prophecies, in
child-rearing, 146–152
Self-image
in adolescence, 107–108
eating behavior and, 151
See also Body-image
Sex therapy, 188–189
Sexual problems
overeating and, *see* Genital
cluster overeaters
physical movements and,
162–165

Society
  attitudes toward obesity,
    154–155
  and changes in attitudes
    about food, 155–156,
    201–202
  child-feeding customs of,
    135–137, 152–154
  encouragement of
    overeating by, 137–139
  Momism and eating
    patterns of, 142–146
  provision of food by,
    134–135
  subcultural attitudes
    toward eating in,
    140–142
Socioeconomic class, obesity
  and, 154–155
Stein-Leventhal syndrome,
  obesity and, 25
Steroid production, obesity
  and, 24–25
Stress
  overeating and, 16, 116, 136,
    200–201
  pheochromocytoma and,
    27–28
  sympathetic nervous
    system's response to,
    28–32
Subcultures, eating patterns
  of, 140–142
Sugar, storage of, 21–22
Sympathetic nervous system
  evaluation under stress,
    29–32
  overeating and, 32
  weight loss and, 28

Tension, physical signs of,
  160–161
  See also Stress
Thermogenesis. *See*
  Diet-induced
  thermogenesis
Thyroid hormone, in
  children, 23–24
Toilet training. *See* Anal
  cluster overeaters
Treatment for overeating
  and adolescent onset,
    194–197
  and adult onset, 198–201
  and anal cluster, 182–187
  and genital cluster, 187–194
  and oral cluster, 178–182
  and social factors, 201–202

Weight control, sympathetic
  nervous system and, 28
Weight gain
  and force feeding in
    nonobese subjects,
    31–32
  and size and number of fat
    cells, 39–40
  and sympathetic response
    under stress, 28–32
Weight loss
  growth hormone and, 33
  pheochromocytoma and,
    28
  See also Anorexia nervosa;
    Dieting
Women. *See* Career women;
  Housewives; Mother-child
  relations; Motherhood